Two Women 1 Disease

A Three Year Memoir

Written by both patient and caregiver of a mother and daughter as they struggle with life, love, survival and lessons learned along the way.

Beth Pauulinch
and
Carol 'CJ' Johnson

Copyright © 2018 by Beth Pauvlinch

All rights reserved. No part of this publication may be reproduced, distributed or transmitted in any form or by any means, including photocopying, recording, or other electronic or mechanical methods, without the prior written permission of the publisher, except in the case of brief quotations embodied in critical reviews and certain other noncommercial uses permitted by copyright law. For permission requests, write to the publisher, addressed "Attention: Permissions Coordinator," at the address below.

Library of Congress Control Number: 2018905238

Beth Pauvlinch Publishing
Beth@ArtbyBeth.com

Cover photo by Beth Pauvlinch
Cover design by Fred Daunno

Ordering Information:
Quantity sales. Special discounts are available on quantity purchases by corporations, associations, and others. For details, contact the "Special Sales Department" at the address above.

Printed and bound in the United States of America

Two Women 1 Disease/ Beth Pauvlinch & Carol 'CJ' Johnson. -- 1st ed.
ISBN 978-0-9995590-0-0

This book was inspired by
Carol Johnson
*My Mother, My Best Friend, My Hero
And Co-Author*

It is my honor to present the world with this book of complete bravery. Every one of the women whom I've had the pleasure to meet throughout this journey has touched my life in a way they will never know! It was the most humbling experience I could have ever traveled.

If this book touches just one soul and makes a difference for them, then I will feel truly blessed.

FOREWORD

FC...that pretty much sums it up. Although my medical career has been relatively short, I've seen too many lives affected by this devastating diagnosis. Reading through Carol and Beth's book, so many of the raw emotions of their experience come forward: Anger, sadness, frustration, terror, strength, and hope. For those looking for answers about dealing with loss, I'm not sure there will ever be an easy fix. All I can say is follow Carol and Beth's path of letting the raw emotions out- bottling up these emotions does not solve anything. Letting them out can be therapeutic. Clearly, the most obvious word that is evident throughout this memoir would be LOVE. I hope this book lets you know that you are not the first person to go through this and take Carol and Beth's lead of sticking together with LOVE.
F*** CANCER
'Dr. S'

–John V. Kiluk, MD FACS
MOFFITT CANCER CENTER

Contents

2009 January 1

Our Cancer (2009-01-15 19:52) – Beth 1
My Cancer (2009-01-18 15:29) – CJ 2
So stinkin' cute . . . (2009-01-18 23:51) – Beth 4
Girls' Day (2009-01-20 23:51) - CJ 6
Tears, tears and more tears! (2009-01-24 09:10) - CJ 7
Button Eyes (2009-01-25 22:52) – Beth 10
Rough Evening (2009-01-29 00:18) - Beth 11

2009 February 13

My parents' dresser! (2009-02-02 16:45) - CJ 13
Being Honest! (2009-02-04 00:22) - Beth 13
Dr. Doogie (2009-02-06 20:20) - CJ 15
People who need people... (2009-02-08 14:30) - CJ 18
Charles Dickens (2009-02-08 23:41) - Beth 20
Are You Listening? (2009-02-10 20:06) - Beth 20
Who knew cancer was a full-time job? (2009-02-12 21:40) - CJ 22
I knew you were there! (2009-02-12 23:20) - Beth 24
'Don't be nice to me!' (2009-02-16 10:07) - CJ 25
Good news, bad news (2009-02-19 10:57) - CJ 27
Update (2009-02-24 10:16) - CJ 29
You can't judge a book by its cover . . . (2009-02-25 12:21) - Beth 30
project 'I am Beautiful' (2009-02-25 17:00) - Beth 32
On a lighter note... (2009-02-26 17:10) - CJ 32

2009 March 37

Chemo Cocktail (2009-03-03 09:37) - CJ 37
What Cancer Cannot Do (2009-03-06 16:41) - CJ 40
Oprah called . . . (2009-03-06 21:06) - Beth 41
More 'angels' (2009-03-08 11:57) - CJ 42
Adding Comments (2009-03-08 16:16) - Beth 44
Girls' Night Out (2009-03-09 22:21) - CJ 44
Miss Hayley (2009-03-09 22:49) - CJ 45
She's so cute! (2009-03-10 00:01) - Beth 46
Mom thanked us today . . . (2009-03-12 20:20) - Beth 48
More issues than Playboy! (2009-03-13 23:59) - CJ 50

Chemo Kicker (2009-03-16 13:45) - Beth 51
Capturing the facts . . . (2009-03-17 00:39) - Beth 53
But Dude, that's not even my church! (2009-03-18 01:00) - CJ 55
No more bad hair days! (2009-03-20 18:24) - CJ 57
Post-op Appointment (2009-03-24 22:39) - Beth 58
3rd Chemo Treatment and Counting . . .   (2009-03-26 23:25) - Beth 60

2009 April 61

You're not going to believe this! (2009-04-01 18:27) - Beth 61
Feeling Helpless (2009-04-02 00:31) - Beth 62
Do you smell that? (2009-04-04 08:00) - CJ 63
Truth be told . . . I ache (2009-04-05 03:14) - Beth 66
Feeling Better (2009-04-05 23:55) - CJ 67
Thanks Janny! (2009-04-09 22:40) - Beth 68
The Last 'Red Devil' (2009-04-12 06:11) - CJ 69
Another side effect (2009-04-15 07:12) - CJ 70
More 'thank you's' (2009-04-18 09:28) - CJ 71
Wow . . . almost two weeks (2009-04-22 00:31) - Beth 72
New chemo (2009-04-24 09:33) - CJ 73
Dreams really do come true! (2009-04-30 18:59) - Beth 74

2009 May 77

Apologies (2009-05-09 07:45) - CJ 77
I promise myself (2009-05-11 22:40) - Beth 78
Hyatt 365 free nights (2009-05-12 14:04) - Beth 79
"drive-through" mastectomies (2009-05-13 02:01) - Beth 81
I spoke too soon! (2009-05-13 11:51) - CJ 81
Pre-Op Appointment (2009-05-15 22:27) - Beth 81
An Epiphany (2009-05-20 16:18) - Beth 82
Taxol, be damned! (2009-05-22 09:19) - CJ 82
The Vine . . . (2009-05-28 21:28) - Beth 83
. . . three things (2009-05-28 22:38) - CJ 84
A Small Price to Pay . . . (2009-05-31 00:11) - Beth 87

2009 June 89

My posse ROCKS!!! (2009-06-04 21:06) - CJ 89
Don't mess with a momma's cub! (2009-06-11 21:45) - Beth 92
Bits 'n Pieces (2009-06-18 19:11) - CJ 93
Appointment updates (2009-06-26 11:32) - CJ 94

2009 July 99

Benefit for Mom (2009-07-06 23:37) - Beth 99

Mom's a CHAMP!! (2009-07-08 23:11) - Beth 101
Cross 'surgery' off the list! (2009-07-13 10:06) - CJ 104
I'M A SURVIVOR!!! (2009-07-15 10:31) - CJ 106
Glad/Sad (2009-07-19 11:06) - CJ... 107
Doc update (2009-07-27 12:05) - CJ... 108
Things I Have Learned from Cancer (so far) (2009-07-28 20:08) - CJ 110

2009 August 113

Long time, no blog! (2009-08-14 17:55) - CJ 113
When it rains..... (2009-08-14 18:20) - CJ.. 114
13 Down, 20 to Go! (2009-08-23 21:16) - CJ................................... 117

2009 September 119

And the winner is... (2009-09-12 11:25) - CJ 119

2009 October 121

Long Overdue Update (2009-10-06 12:07) – CJ 121
Doc's appointment (2009-10-21 17:25) - CJ.................................... 123
The BEST Surgeon in the World!!! (2009-10-25 09:19) - CJ 124
A Heartfelt Apology! (2009-10-28 07:23) - Beth 125
Thank you, God! (2009-10-28 10:20) - CJ.. 126

2009 November 129

NOW I believe it !! (2009-11-08 16:06) - CJ.................................... 129
Feeling better! (2009-11-22 08:31) - CJ.. 130
I am SO THANKFUL.... (2009-11-26 07:33) - CJ............................... 131
Thank you, Mom! (2009-11-26 09:23) - Beth.................................. 132

2009 December 133

Thank you, Bethie! (2009-12-09 20:02) - CJ 133

2010 February 135

Update: (2010-02-23 21:29) - Beth 135

2010 March 137

Thanks, Big Guy!!! (2010-03-03 12:34) - CJ..................................... 137
Old friends and new boobs (2010-03-07 09:44) - CJ 137

2010 April 143

Bad day at Black Rock (2010-04-19 15:55) - CJ 143

2010 May 145

Doc update (2010-05-07 16:24) - CJ... 145

    Beth's photography (2010-05-08 15:44) - CJ 146

2010 July 147

    Happy, happy.... (2010-07-08 12:04) - CJ 147

2010 August 149

    Doc Update (2010-08-13 22:06) - CJ 149
    Call from Dr. O (2010-08-15 21:21) - Beth 150
    Round 2: Me - 1, Cancer -2 (2010-08-19 17:01) - CJ 151
    Not Again!!! (2010-08-19 22:40) - Beth 152
    The Ultimate Optimist Turns Realist (2010-08-31 18:47) - Beth........ 155

2010 September 159

    Gotta' take the bad with the good! (2010-09-01 22:52) - CJ 159
    Pancreatic cancer deserves HAZARD PAY!!! (2010-09-02 19:50) - CJ 160
    One week down (2010-09-10 13:09) - CJ 162
    3 am??? (2010-09-13 20:45) - Beth 163
    '...but you're in such good health, otherwise.' (2010-09-15 09:15) - CJ
    165
    NOW what?? (2010-09-17 15:21) - CJ.. 166
    Weekly report (2010-09-24 06:41) - CJ 167
    Neupogen Shots (2010-09-28 10:51) - CJ....................................... 169
    Potentially GREAT news!! (2010-09-28 20:48) - Beth 169
    PS . . . (2010-09-28 21:26) - Beth 172
    How do I really feel? (2010-09-29 18:33) - Beth 172

2010 October 175

    When God closes a door... (2010-10-01 12:56) - CJ......................... 175
    Thanks, girls!! (2010-10-03 15:11) - CJ.. 176
    Chemo week (2010-10-07 13:09) - CJ 177
    Odds and ends (2010-10-09 18:41) - CJ 178
    Good news (2010-10-12 10:56) - CJ 180
    Fond memories (2010-10-22 17:31) - CJ.. 181
    As I Sit Here . . . (2010-10-27 22:34) - Beth.................................... 183
    If I'm doing better why am I feeling worse? (2010-10-28 10:02) - CJ 184

2010 November 185

    UNCLE!!! (2010-11-15 21:39) - Beth 185
    Just things I think about . . . (2010-11-18 20:18) - Beth 186
    An Emotional Thanksgiving! (2010-11-23 19:37) - Beth 187
    Happy Thanksgiving! (2010-11-25 21:41) - CJ................................. 188

2010 December 191

I Ache For Her . . . (2010-12-06 20:58) - Beth 191
Freeing . . . (2010-12-11 21:25) - Beth 192
. . . without my Mother! (2010-12-23 23:55) - Beth 193
...without my Daughter! (2010-12-24 10:03) - CJ 194

2011 January 197

The Holidays . . . (2011-01-03 22:20) - Beth 197
I can't seem to stop crying . . . (2011-01-04 21:49) - Beth 199
Platelet Transfusion . . . (2013-08-25 18:39) - Beth 200
It dawned on me . . . (2011-01-26 20:42) - Beth 202

2011 February 205

And The Nominees Are . . . (2011-02-08 19:42) - Beth 205

2011 April 207

Spending time with family . . . (2011-04-02 22:49) - Beth 207

2011 May 209

I don't call, I don't write... (2011-05-06 23:19) - CJ 209

2011 June 211

Wow, a lot has happened . . . (2011-06-06 18:35) - Beth 211
All Her Angels . . . (2011-06-26 19:32) - Beth 212

2011 July 215

Let's catch up . . . (2011-07-10 17:53) - Beth 215

2011 August 219

Not a good Monday! (2011-08-08 10:10) - Beth 219

2011 November 221

MUCH NEEDED UPDATE (2011-11-05 08:50) - Beth 221
Your Re-Birth (2011-11-07 01:07) - Beth 222
And the process gets uglier . . . (2011-11-11 22:24) - Beth 224
Terminal Restlessness Over . . . (2011-11-13 12:52) - Beth 227
Now What? (2011-11-18 21:05) - Beth 231
Unresponsive (2011-11-19 19:45) - Beth 232
Spread your wings and fly, my angel! (2011-11-20 18:32) - Beth 234
Grieving . . . (2011-11-21 17:57) - Beth 234
Seriously . . . (2011-11-29 21:01) - Beth 235

2011 December 237

Ma's Remains . . . (2011-12-01 17:55) - Beth 237

And life goes on . . . (2011-12-05 20:57) - Beth 240
Heeeeeeeeere's Janny... (2011-12-15 08:55) - Janice...................... 241
Happy Birthday, My Angel! (2011-12-19 20:27) - Beth...................... 243
The Eulogy (2011-12-19 20:48) - Beth 246
Christmas without her . . . (2011-12-26 20:13) - Beth 251
From Bad Day to Sad Day (2011-12-29 20:49) - Beth 255
Dear 2011, (2011-12-30 19:10) - Beth 257

2012 January 261

I especially miss her today . . . (2012-01-05 19:43) - Beth 261
'Today I am grateful . . . ' (2012-01-08 19:26) - Beth 262
Bursting with Excitement . . . (2012-01-10 19:38) - Beth 267
Her Car's gone now . . . (2012-01-16 19:11) - Beth 269
Only two more days . . . (2012-01-18 18:24) - Beth 270
End of This Chapter . . . (2012-01-22 21:41) - Beth 271

2012 August 273

One final sentiment . . . (2012-08-25 18:34) - Beth 273

2009 January

Our Cancer (2009-01-15 19:52) – Beth

On November 17th of 2008, my mother confessed to me that she has breast cancer. She 'confessed' as if it were her fault. As if she was guilty of something. Seems silly, I know. She is pretty silly . . . and short too! Oh, and don't get offended, but we tease each other a lot, but it is all in a joking manner. You gotta laugh just to get through life (and because it's fun!) Sometimes when you're sad, it makes it harder not to cry when someone is being nice to you. Don't you agree? So, whenever we're on the verge of tears and we don't want to cry, we'll say, "Don't be nice to me." Which usually ends in name calling and then we laugh and we don't want to cry anymore. Pure genius, we are!!

She's my mom. She's my best friend. She's my inspiration. She's my biggest fan. She's my world and my whole heart! I really don't know what I will do without her. She lives and works with me. She is the first person I see in the morning and the last person I see before going to sleep.

I'm guessing you're starting to understand how close my mom & I are . . . now I can continue.

Anyway, since we never want to burden the other with our own feelings when we know that the other person is dealing with emotions as well, we hold them in. That's not good. You know that what goes in . . . eventually, has to come out. We can learn to let it out in a calm and responsible, yet productive manner rather than go on a spree of stomping on everyone's toes that came a little too close to our own.

I talked with her about creating a blog where we can just release our emotions and have a place where we can feel comfortable getting things off our chest (no pun intended). We agreed and so it begins. We welcome any type of interactivity, so, if you have something to say . . . by all means, please feel free.

I guess this will be the beginning of 'Two Women ~ 1 Disease . . . This is our journey' Let the journey begin.

> John Pauvlinch (2009-01-20 17:30:00)
> I know this is your blog to post your feelings, but let me be the first to comment.
> Carol, I cannot pretend to understand what you are going through. But I want to say that I am very proud of you for, not only how you are handling it mentally, but what you are doing to beat it instead of letting it beat you.
> Beth, you are quite an impressive daughter. Your devotion to your Mother is an inspiration to all children out there today.
> I am very proud of both of you and I am here if I can do anything to help or just make things easier for either of you. I love you both.
> John

My Cancer (2009-01-18 15:29) – CJ

She's my daughter. She's my best friend. She's my inspiration. She gives meaning to my life I have no reason to expect. She's my world and my whole heart. She's the first person I hug in the morning and the last person I hug at night. I can't bear the thought of leaving her! And I guess that's the reason I have decided to 'take' this journey.

On April 14, 2007, as I sat on the couch watching tv, I reached down to scratch my right breast and felt a huge lump. It was so huge, in fact, that I couldn't imagine why I hadn't felt this in the shower. It actually seemed to have appeared overnight.

I immediately 'put my head in the sand'. If I didn't acknowledge it, it wasn't there. My daughter already had so much stress in her life that I just didn't feel I could burden her with anymore. So for the next 19 months, I kept it to myself. It didn't seem to be growing or changing in any way until June 2008, (shortly after the deaths of my mother and a brother) when I noticed that the nipple had inverted and had begun to discharge a light-yellowish fluid. The skin was puckered and rather 'burned' looking. And still, I ignored it. I had done some internet research and deduced that it was probably inflammatory breast cancer, a rare and particularly aggressive type.

In November 2008, we lost a friend to cancer and I began to panic. I knew I needed to tell someone, even though I had decided long ago that I was 'going with all my parts'! I watched my dear, dear grandmother lose the battle with breast and bone cancer back in the 70's and determined then that I would never go through that. It was a losing battle! But at the very least, my daughter, sister and nieces needed to know that this horrible disease was closer to them than 'grandmother/great-grandmother'.

I gathered every bit of nerve I could to tell my daughter on November 17, 2008, and two days later, told my sister and brothers. They were all supportive even though some of them did not agree with my decision not to have treatment.

I was beginning to have some pain from it and had no health insurance, so after speaking with several resources decided it would be best to visit the emergency room, at the very least to find someone who could/would help with pain management down the road.

Since then, lots of tears, lots of testing, appointments with doctors, social workers, agencies, etc., (and much more to come), yes, it is cancer, but from the information they have at this point, probably not inflammatory. I am not a candidate for a lumpectomy because of the location and size of the tumor. What I have to 'look forward' to is a mastectomy, chemotherapy, radiation, hormone therapy. Sounds like fun, huh?

I have decided to go ahead with the treatment because I CAN'T bear the thought of leaving my daughter, although I dread what is ahead. The 'powers that be' continue to tell us how much progress has been made, but to me, it seems that cancer always wins!

I know there are survivors and have actually talked with several, but that doesn't take away the fear. I seem to be fine one minute and the next, being reduced to tears. I just don't seem to be able to deal with it. I know the pride is a big part of it. And even though I continue to hear my dad's voice, 'Pride goeth before a fall, little girl', just can't shake it. It does terrible things to your self-esteem, especially if you don't have much, to begin with!

My daughter and my sister go to all my appointments with me and, bless their hearts, are so patient with my moods and tears! My siblings and friends continue to support me and are all very glad that I have decided to be treated.

And so, the journey continues.

So stinkin' cute . . . (2009-01-18 23:51) – Beth

Last week after meeting with one of the 'survivors', we went to the wig shop. Mom was getting discouraged initially, but then we found one (completely out of her norm!) and we both loved it!! She looks so stinkin' cute! She walked in a spikey redhead and walked out a straight brunette. I like to see her go back to her roots (that was funny!). Anyway, I'll try to talk her into posting a photo in her wig. I can pretty much talk her into anything. One time on vacation, I talked her into putting buttons on her eyes. Why? I don't know. Seemed like the thing to do at the time. Turns out, I was right. We laughed while we had button eyes until we cried. It was fun. You should try it sometime and then report back.

Do you know what else has been so special to me during this difficult time? Every night before we go to bed, we go to 'The Memory Vase' and read aloud a memory that we've had together. We have had so many wonderful times together! For those of you that don't know, 'The Memory Vase' was originally created for my mother about five years ago as a Christmas gift. At the time, she lived many miles away from me so I wanted her to have a way to reflect on the many memories we have to share with each other whenever she was missing me. I don't know, but somehow, with enough comments about marketing this as a product, I've done just that. I'm not here to sell products, just trying to give you some background details on who we are and what we do. Anyway, that has been a very special time for us both to look forward to.

Mom and I held an outside conference today and came up with our next vision. I think it will be a very positive situation to be in during this particular time in our lives and could possibly be very positive to others, as well. I can't tell ya much more than that because I don't know if y'all can be trusted (just kidding, kinda), but stay tuned ... I will be revealing little by little.

Anonymous (2009-01-19 19:44:00)
Not sure what to say (1st time I have ever blogged) other than I love you both

and you will have my support throughout your journey (which I am so glad you decided to take). Mike

Girls' Day (2009-01-20 23:51) - CJ

First of all, it was about 12 years ago, not five, that I received 'The Memory Vase' as a gift. Precisely why we actually NEED 'The Memory Vase'!! And it has become one of the highlights of my day, as well. We only put good memories in it so they always make us laugh. And she really did make me put buttons on my eyes. We have pictures to prove it!! We also did it with matchbooks! Hey, ya' gotta' make your own fun!

We'll be having a 'girls' day' on Thursday. Not your typical 'shopping, lunch, movie girls' day'. This one will be at the hospital. I will be having a bone scan as well as CAT scans of the liver, lungs and pelvis. My sister will be having mammograms and ultrasounds (precautionary) and my daughter will be our cheerleader! Apparently, I will be having a dye injection for breakfast and two very large bottles of contrast liquid for lunch. Not what I had in mind for girls' day. I was really hoping for a big, fat cheeseburger!

> Janice (2009-01-22 05:58:00)
> I, too, was hoping for a cheeseburger, or a chicken sandwich - even better. I'm very nervous about today. I think I'll probably feel guilty if my mammo and ultrasound are okay. (You can take the girl out of the Catholic Church but you can't take the Catholic Church out of the girl.) I know that Carol would never want me to feel that way and would be crushed if they were to come back positive, as was I when I got the news about her cancer. It's really hard for me to say that word when I'm talking about her. This is my Louie, for crying out loud, what would I do without her?!? But I am optimistic and so thankful that she's decided to have treatment. All of this has been very hard on all of us, but my heart breaks every time I think of what she and Beth must be feeling. I wish there was more I could do, but for now, I'll just be there for them, until they throw me out.

Tears, tears and more tears! (2009-01-24 09:10) - CJ

We kind of went from telling my family about a lump to a positive biopsy result as if it were one step. Believe me, it was much more. I really was fine as long as I had my blinders on, but once I told my family, it was a different story. For some reason, once it was out in the open it felt like a death sentence. I began dreaming of deceased family members and friends every single night. And the really weird part of that is that when I relocated ten years ago to be near my daughter, my dreams, which had always been in glorious technicolor and very detailed, completely stopped! Now they had begun again and were constant reminders that life does not go on forever. I cried constantly, day and night and my daughter had to bear the brunt of all this. Even our little dog picked up on the mood around the house and became mopey and whiney and laid outside my bedroom door. She would always run to wake me when she heard me having a nightmare and if she couldn't get in, would carry on till my daughter brought her in to see me.

The emergency room visit, which started the whole process, lasted six hours. They did blood work, a chest x-ray, mammograms of both breasts and ultrasound of the right and recommended an ultrasound of the left. The medicine they gave me to calm me for the expected pain of the mammogram (because the mass is so large – 6.6 x 5.7 x 3.5 cm) made me sick as a dog. But at least the mammogram ended up being completely painless.

I had already told (through tears) everyone with whom I came in contact that I was not having treatment and they said I still had to have a doctor for pain management down the road. They referred me to a surgeon who I visited two days later, and whose bedside manner was not only non-existent but who was downright rude. We waited 90 minutes in his office and he gave us 90 seconds of his time before he pushed me back on the table and announced that he would be doing a biopsy and left the office, not even giving us a chance to ask any questions. When he and his entourage came back in with their little bag of goodies, I asked what this biopsy was going to tell us and he said it would tell us what type of cancer this was (he thought it looked like inflammatory) and how to best treat it. When I reiterated that I didn't want treatment, and what the emergency room had told me, he turned on his heel, told his resident to give me a referral and walked out. I understand that he deals with this all day, every day, but it's all new to us. A little compassion would have been nice. We left his office vowing never to go back, me in tears!

'Dr. Rude' had given me a referral to an oncologist since 'this office doesn't DO pain management'. I made an appointment with the new doctor and everyone that I spoke with told me they were going to take care of me and were sincere.

I am lucky enough to have in my city a free breast and cervical cancer screening program with lots of resources for women with no insurance. They actually found me, apparently through my visit to the emergency room, and I was enrolled in the program. I spoke (she spoke, I cried) with a survivor whose mother is also a survivor and who runs a program which guides women through the process and helps in so many different ways. They have a program that helps with up to $500 per person for medicines, transportation to appointments, even wigs. They have get-togethers to teach women creative ways to apply makeup and to tie scarves, things to keep up self-esteem, as well as dealing with the whole issue of cancer.

I met with another survivor, a nurse practitioner, (and cried) who works with the program and whose daughter and sister are also survivors. There I had a pap smear and lots of discussion about the whole experience and how important it is to stay positive.

By the time I met with the doctor you would think I wouldn't have any tears left. Not so. Believe me, I still have plenty! And what a difference! From the time we stepped into his office, everyone we came into contact with treated us with dignity and respect. The doctor actually sat down with us for an hour and a half before he even examined me. He listened to all my concerns (through tears), he answered all the questions we had and some we hadn't thought of. He talked about how things have changed, and continue to change, as far as treatment. He said he felt like he was almost two years behind trying to treat this and wanted to get going quickly. He wanted to do bone, liver, lung and pelvis scans to see if it had traveled. He felt that some chemo to try to shrink it, a mastectomy, more chemo, radiation, and hormones were the way to go, but first, we needed a biopsy, to which I finally agreed.

The biopsy, even after three Xanax and a local, hurt like hell! Since the biopsy was positive, 'an infiltrating ductal type of intermediate grade, 70 % hormone positive', I qualify for a special Medicaid program for breast and cervical cancer, thank goodness, which pays for all this testing and surgery, including reconstruction! Because it is hormone positive, I am already on Femara and will receive Herceptin with the chemo. However, we will forgo the chemo beforehand and go straight to the surgery. I am currently awaiting a call from the hospital where the surgery will be performed.

Next step, scans. After a bone scan and CAT scans of the liver, lungs and pelvis, they determined they needed a static of my right femur and x-rays of my spine and right leg. Not sure why, but apparently my doc will have the results in a few days and I will find out. I actually thought I would get through this appointment without tears, but I was wrong. When they told me they needed the additional x-rays, it scared me. Has it spread? I'm trying to stay positive, but I learned from a master. We used to tease my mom that if she had nothing to worry about, she would make things up!!

For all who are following this blog, thank you so much for your kind words, prayers and support! And James, you goon. Save a little of that Catholic guilt for me!! We'll never throw you out!!

Button Eyes (2009-01-25 22:52) – Beth

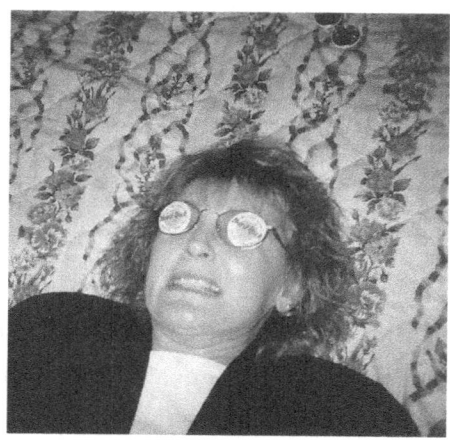

Oh, you're going to love this. My mom actually found the photo of her with buttons on her eyes and agreed to let me post it. I took it in a London hotel in December 1996. I was working on a job in Boston and called a radio station for a contest and won a trip to London. Of course, I took my mom with me. We had a blast! One of my most memorable moments was when we were getting ready to go out for the day. She had showered and was preparing to curl her hair. All of sudden she yelled 'my hair's on fire and the curling iron is melting!' She hadn't thought that they have 220 plugs there and you needed an adapter to use these things. Maybe you had to be there, but we still laugh really hard over that! We didn't find the matchbook pictures yet but will post them upon finding them. We had a decent weekend. Mom is definitely doing better with her positive attitude. We watched an Extreme Home Makeover the other day and she started feeling guilty about feeling sad and mad over this when there are people out there dealing with so much more. This particular show had an 8-year-old boy who had brittle bone disease. He had, during his lifetime, broken every bone in his body. To see this little boy was to love him. And he was just the most positive little one you could ever meet! I took both my girls to the park the other day to get out into the sunshine and get a little bit of exercise. It was nice. Of course, Roxy kept us laughing. She is so silly. We told her when we got her that making us laugh was her only job and she does just that!

Rough Evening (2009-01-29 00:18) - Beth

I'm hanging in, but tonight is not really a good night for me. Mom's scans came back in a not so positive light. We were worried when they requested additional scans and X-Rays of her inner thigh. So, results are that there is a concern in her right thigh. The doctor thought it was unusual for only one bone to be affected, so I have to hope that whatever they're finding is not associated with cancer. That it's just some weird thing that isn't damaging to her health. I HAVE to be the one to keep the hope alive!! Right?!

Sometimes, I just wanna break, but I know I can't. Part of me doesn't want to type this cause I don't want to burden my mom with my feelings when I can't even imagine what she must be going through in her mind. And the other part does because it is about being honest, right? This is hurting me!! It's tearing me apart! I hate seeing my mom in so much pain, both emotionally & physically. I feel useless. I want to take this pain away from her and protect her. I can't do that and it kills me. As much as I try to make her believe that we are in this together, she has to know that it is HER attitude that is going to bring her through this. I can be her 'rock', I can be her everything, but she has to 'BELIEVE'!! I love her so much!

2009 February

My parents' dresser! (2009-02-02 16:45) - CJ

My appointment with the surgeon is this Thursday, 2/5, and I am getting very nervous. I have picked up copies of all my scans, mammos, x-rays, reports, etc., and am working my way through the myriad of paperwork that has to be completed by then.

For someone who has been to the doctor's <u>once</u> in the last ten years (for a cut finger which required 11 stitches or I wouldn't have gone then, either!), it is quite disconcerting to have appointments at least once a week, usually more! Not to mention, barely more than an Advil or two for ten years and the top of my dresser now looks like my parents' dresser used to look! Pills to go to sleep, pills for pain, more pills for pain, hormones, vitamins . . . is the cure worse than the disease?!!

Because of the 'area of concern' in my right thigh, my doc has ordered a PET scan for February 9. I will see him again on February 12 and he will, hopefully, have good news for us about that.

Being Honest! (2009-02-04 00:22) - Beth

It's so funny, not ha-ha funny, but weird funny that everyone involved with the appointments, even the blogging is concerned about what everyone else is thinking. We are so concerned with hurting other people's feelings that we don't even want to honor our own. We keep talking with each other and speaking of the ridiculousness of the situation that it is almost comical. Like a freakin' Seinfeld episode or something. When are we going to speak from the heart? C'mon, speak up!! I'm going to do it from now on!

And let me start by saying that we received a wonderful gift from a brother of my mom's. He sent my mom a 'handwritten letter' which she couldn't remember him ever doing before with a $100 dollar bill wrapped in it. He told her to fill the gas tank and take 'the girls' to lunch. It was so much appreciated!!

Another family member (second cousin . . . weirdo, why does that offend you?), sent the link to one of my published books to EVERYONE he knows and made quite a few sales from it. I'm pretty sure he made most of the sales!! Thanks, Mike!

Funny thing is, we were wondering if we should mention the nice gestures people were gracing us with for fear that we might offend someone. As I type this, the thoughts ponder in my head . . . how could a nice gesture possibly offend anyone? I guess it's just ridiculous thinking, is all.

I took a break from the blog long enough to hold my mom's hand. I held it for a long time, but it just doesn't seem long enough. I held it until my hand went numb, but I know that when she is gone . . . I am going to miss that 'numb' feeling and wish that I had more time. And I also know that I'm going to experience even more 'numb' than I ever thought possible.

I remember a long time ago when I was so 'distressed' when my Grandfather was tickling me so much, it actually hurt. And I remember trying desperately, to release myself from his grip. Then I remember him passing and not having his strong arms to hold me tight and protect me. Bastard, how could he make me feel so safe and then abandon me? I just don't want these feelings to come out with my mom. I don't want to have any regrets!!

I believe in my heart of hearts that she is going to pull through this. It is going to be a tough road, but we will get through it. All of this just reminds me that we are all mortal and we will all die one day . . . and for whatever reason, I don't want to live without her!!

> Anonymous (2009-02-04 11:25:00)
> We are thinking of you every day and wishing we could just give you a big hug. And also be there to help out in any way. We love you so much and pray that you will soon be healed, remember miracles do happen. Hopefully, we will be able to come down this month and we can sit and laugh for a bit.
> Love, Andy, Heidi, Hayley and Cayden

> Anonymous (2009-02-04 16:30:00)
> This is so great, and for you to talk not even about what is going on just your feelings speaks volumes to everyone who reads this. We love you all and know that this is a tough time so whatever you feel, feel it, people do nice gestures because YOU deserve it and they know that it will never be taken for granted. You have to let people help you too because for some that is how they talk it out and otherwise deal with feelings they have. Whatever happens, you have a great support system and many, many prayers are being said daily for you and the road might be tough, but my bets are on you women cause you are some strong contenders.
> Love You! Lisa

Dr. Doogie (2009-02-06 20:20) - CJ

I have been very jittery all week worrying about the surgeon's appointment. Worrying and being jittery makes me clumsy (clumsier than normal!) and on Wednesday, I banged my fourth toe on my right foot, painfully, on the desk. By early evening, it was swollen and just about every color of the rainbow. Not bad enough, I did it again and this time it brought me to tears! I'm pretty sure I got it right this time because I think it's broken. I iced it down and taped it, but it's not getting any better. The stupid thing ('stupider' than doing it twice) is that my third toe has been numb for several months (I've diagnosed myself as having peripheral neuropathy!), so why couldn't it have been the one that's numb?!! Right, what fun would that be? Yesterday I had my appointment with the surgeon. What a difference! 'Dr. Rude' definitely needs to go back to school for Bedside Manner 101, or better yet, take lessons from Dr. Doogie! I only call him that because he looks like he's about 12! Actually, we'll call him Dr. Surgeon just so we don't get him confused with Dr. Oncologist. He walked into the room with his arms wide open, literally, and said, 'You get a hug' to which I replied, 'Great, just don't hurt my boob!' And he proceeded to give me a huge bear hug.

He sat down with 'the girls' and me, after introducing himself to them, and the first thing he told me is that the one thing I need to remember is that he will be at my side every step of the way! WOW, what a way to instill confidence! He gave us a rundown on cancer, complete with drawings, and some of the treatments I will be facing without once reprimanding me for waiting so long. He said that if it is in my bones, there really isn't anything they can do for that but that he knows people who have it and are still going strong after ten years, and of course, the chemo could shrink that as well and keep it localized. He told me that I will have chemo first to try to shrink the tumor, then the mastectomy, more chemo, radiation, and hormones, just as Dr. Oncologist said. As this is a research and teaching hospital, he introduced two residents and asked if I minded if they stayed while he examined me. He was very gentle and explained what he was doing and what he was looking for as he went along, I believe, as much for my sake as for the residents. After the exam, he felt that a sonogram of the sentinel lymph node was necessary. We were ushered into another room for this, I was smeared up with the goop and the sonogram began, after which he decided a needle biopsy was necessary. A little painful, but not as bad as the previous breast biopsy. He told us to come back in 30 minutes and he would have the results rushed.

When we sat down with him again, he said the biopsy was showing all was good, but that he didn't believe it because of the size of the tumor. He wants to do a tissue biopsy, tentatively scheduled for 2/16, so he can be sure what, if any, nodes need to be removed at the time of the mastectomy. At the same time, he will implant a port under my skin on the left side of my chest, which will provide direct entry to my blood system. This will be used to administer the chemo, IVs or draw blood. This allows the drugs to be given slowly, reducing side effects, protects the vein and eliminates extra needle sticks to find a good vein.

He will teleconference with Dr. Oncologist so they can coordinate my treatment and then, I guess, we're off to the races! He said I'm in for a long journey, but reminded me again, that he will be right beside me.

I must say I was relieved at this appointment, not only because Dr. Surgeon is so compassionate, but because it actually buys me some time before the surgery. Don't get me wrong, I'm not looking forward to the chemo and all the crummy effects of that, but the mastectomy is still scarier.

On the way home, the girls and I had dinner. THANKS, Joe!!! We appreciate it more than you know!

Today, Dr. Oncologist's office called to schedule me for a baseline echocardiogram on 2/10. Apparently, in a very small percentage of people (less than 5 %), the efficiency of the heart is affected by the toxicity of the combination of the drugs used in chemo. The echocardiogram will be repeated every 12 weeks for a year to be sure no changes are taking place.

I'm thinking of changing my address to that of the hospital! Stay tuned, lots more to come!

People who need people... (2009-02-08 14:30) - CJ

For whatever reason, it has always been very difficult for my daughter and me to ask for, and/or accept, help. Probably why my dad always told me, 'Pride goeth before a fall, little girl'!! In my case, I want to be independent, self-sufficient, strong, and in my mind, if I have to ask for help, I become dependent, needy and weak. Not other people, just me. Crazy, I know, but old habits die hard. In my daughter's case, not one of the better things she learned from me. A perfect example of a case where an instruction manual for raising children would have certainly come in handy!! Sorry, sweetie!!

We are so blessed to have such a great support group of family and friends. We have received so many kind words, cards, letters, and prayers.

First and foremost, what would I do without my precious daughter?!! She has been my rock, beside me every step of the way with a positive outlook, even though there are times, I'm sure when she feels unable to face it. With all the other stress she is under, she manages to boost me up when I feel down, whether it's with jokes, with a stern lecture or just sitting quietly holding my hand. She spends her time driving me to and from appointments and hanging out in doctors' offices and hospitals. Not much fun! I thank God every day for her! Thank you and I love you more than you know, sweetheart!

On Christmas day, Beth and I decided that we just wanted to spend the day in our jammies, alone with our little dog, 'being thankful'. That afternoon the doorbell rang. We weren't expecting anyone and peeped out to see a package on the doorstep. Inside was a toy for the dog, a grocery store gift certificate, a box of candy and two cards, one for each of us, from our friends, Harry, Rachel, and Chris. I opened mine and immediately burst into tears. Out fell three $100 bills! Inside was written, 'You are our Christmas Carol. Please take a mini-vacation on us.' My first response was, 'I can't accept this, this is just too much!' Apparently, they had already told Beth that it was something they wanted to do. And I still cry when I think or talk about it! 'Thank you' just doesn't seem sufficient!

I have received cards from long-ago friends with whom I had lost touch. Thank you all so much for your words of encouragement and support. One was a 22-year cancer survivor and part of her message said that when things look the darkest, to whisper the name 'Jesus' for strength. Thank you, Kathy; I do get strength from it.

My sister, even though she has a job and her own house and family to take care of, goes to all my appointments with us. An extra pair of ears, a source of questions we don't think of (she thinks she's a doctor!), support for both of us and, of course, comic relief! And yesterday, she even dropped off lunch. Chicken salad and cookies! Thanks, James, it was yummy!! (And by the way, she got good results on her mammograms and sonograms, thank God!!)

Our lawn man gave me a big hug the other day and told me that he put me on the prayer chain at his church so I've got 800 people praying for me! Thanks, Mr. Marshall. I can use all the prayers I can get!

I received the most beautiful hand-written letter from my brother, whose faith and inspirational words are such a comfort to me. And of course, (he's Joey P.!), he also included $100 for gas and lunch for 'the girls' with all these testing trips! Thanks honey. We've already enjoyed one lunch and only wish you could have been there with us!

To my nieces and nephews who send such encouraging emails and comments on the blog, thank you all so much!

My friend, Rick, sent a beautiful card and a check to spend on 'something we need'. Thanks, honey!

My long-time friends follow the blog and check in regularly to see how things are going. Thanks, Bob and Joan. I appreciate your support and encouragement more than you know!

My 'other mother' has put me on the prayer list at her church. Thanks, Mom!

This is, by no means, a complete list of the kindnesses we have received. The fact that so many people have offered their support and help, hopefully, will make it easier for us to reach out, not to feel as though we are 'putting someone out'. So I will try to heed Barbra's words when she sings, "people who need people are the luckiest people in the world'.

I love and appreciate you all so very much!

Charles Dickens (2009-02-08 23:41) - Beth

My goodness hasn't mom become the Charles Dickens in the family? I guess this writing thing is doing her well. She actually just told me earlier today that blogging about all of this is really like therapy. That makes me feel great for her!! She doesn't get out anywhere and the only person that she is around is me, and sometimes Janny. So, I knew she would need some sort of 'outlet' for her frustrations and emotions. There is such a wide range of emotions that you endure while dealing with cancer, as a patient and a caregiver.

Are You Listening? (2009-02-10 20:06) - Beth

I need to talk with the only one I believe can help me now. Just because he/she hasn't signed up as a follower, I think, is still following . . .

Dear God,

It's just me, Beth. You should remember me because you've responded to some of my requests in the past. Some, I thought you ignored, but then realized that maybe you did respond and your answer was just 'No'. My questions these days aren't exactly 'yes or no' answers so I need more information from you if you have a second.

Today was the hardest day for me at the hospital. Mom had to get an Echo to make sure that her heart will handle the chemo alright because it is; after all, poison they will be shooting into her. I sat there and literally watched as my precious mother's heart beat right before my very eyes. I'm guessing it is what a mother feels like watching her new baby's heart beat (which is another bone I have to pick with you, but that's a whole other blog). Yet, it is quite the opposite at the same time because a new mom is celebrating life and I am fearing death. It considerably slows my breathing as I think of her breath ceasing forever. And I can't fight back the tears.

I know that you must be teaching me something, but I'm not seeing it. I'm trying desperately to stay positive but seems like you're fighting me on this. Can you please tell me why? Are you trying to build 'character'? Because ask anyone up there that knows me . . . I have enough 'character'!!

God, I feel like I should be there 110% with my mom dealing with Satan, which I do believe cancer to be. But then we get led back into another 'Great Depression' and now, I have to worry about keeping a roof over my dear mother's head while she is healing? What is going on? Have I done something to just piss you off? Are you listening?

I'm sorry for whatever I've done, and you can choose to forgive me or you can choose to listen to the thousands of other people that are praying to you for my mother's strength, both physically and emotionally. You can't be mad at all of them, too!

Maybe you are not ready, or perhaps, it's not yet time for me to know the answers to all of my questions, but I beg of you . . .

Who knew cancer was a full-time job?
(2009-02-12 21:40) - CJ

What a week! Sunday night I was in a lot of pain. Usually, it's not so bad but this was definitely a '10'. Percocet, two at a time, was not helping, nor was it letting me get any sleep. It continued into Monday when I was scheduled for my PET scan. I fasted for six hours; we got to the hospital, checked in and were taken back to the room when they determined that the equipment was not working. Rescheduled for Wednesday. By the time I got home, I was in unbearable pain. A Vicodin left over from the ER visit in December did the trick. Didn't really help the pain, but allowed me to sleep through it.

Tuesday was relatively little pain and we went for the echocardiogram, totally non-invasive, the kind I don't mind. Except that it was the most traumatic for Beth. She is under so much stress and it breaks my heart to have to put her through more. I wonder if a broken heart shows up on the test. We intended to come home and spend time together with our little dog, but a message from Dr. Surgeon's office thwarted that. Seems they want magnification views of some of the calcifications in my left breast, although I've already had mammograms and sonograms before I come in for my surgery.

Wednesday, fasting for six hours in preparation for the PET scan again. After three attempts (ouch) at inserting the IV, saline was administered, along with an injection of radioactive dye. I rested quietly for about an hour before I was placed on the table, a strap around my feet to hold them together and bundled in blankets. Apparently, the usual scan is 'eyes to thighs', but because of the suspicious spot on my thigh, Dr. O. wanted mine to scan to my knees. After 24 minutes, the test was finished, results in tomorrow.

Thursday, a visit to Dr. O. and some good news, the spot on my thigh did not 'light up' on the PET scan! More good news, the echocardiogram shows that my heart is good! Thanks, Big Guy, and all those who have sent so many prayers our way!! My next appointment is in two weeks when I will begin my first round of chemo. I will have it every two weeks for two months, then round two will begin.

Tonight we attended a support group event. All the women were in fairly advanced stages of treatment. It started off great with a survivor showing wigs and turbans and explaining different types of prostheses, gift bags, door prizes, refreshments, the whole nine yards. It ended up scaring the hell out of me with them all telling me horror stories about the chemo and surgery! HELLO. I thought this was support! I thought for sure I was either going to pass out or throw up all over them! I probably won't be going to that support group again anytime soon.

Friday, mammos at Dr. Surgeon's and my pre-op appointment when I will meet with the anesthesiologist, have blood work and any other testing done.

Saturday and Sunday, gee, two days 'off'. Catch up on all the things around the house that have been pushed to the back burner with all this running to appointments. I don't know how much I'll be able to do after Tuesday. I understand the recovery period is one to two weeks.

I knew you were there! (2009-02-12 23:20) - Beth

Dear God,

Thank you, thank you, thank you, thank you, thank you!! Amen!

I was really trying to plan for the worst and hope for the best today and I was very nervous about getting the results of mom's Echo & PET scans. The news couldn't have been any better! I guess God is following the blog!

She is just adorable and organized on all these appointments. I'm very proud of her that she has taken this on as a mission and she prepares for all three of us. When we got to the doctor's office, she calmly reaches into her little bag that she carries around with her now that she has surrendered her purse because that just wasn't big enough anymore. She keeps her meds and records and whatnot in there. I've started carrying a much larger bag myself with laptop, books, notepads . . . anything I can utilize 'wait time' for 'work time'. Anyway, today she pulled out three notepads, with pens attached to each, and said we all had one if we needed to take notes. She's determined, at this point, I love seeing that passion in her!!

Then, with the good results, I was really looking forward to the 'Support Group'. I've been pushing mom to go, but she's just not very social, by choice. She would rather just stay home. I think it is important for her to talk to people who have been or are going through the same situation as hers. I can be her 'rock' all day long and I can feel similar emotional pain, but I can't possibly take on 'I know how you feel' relating to the physical pain and I think that's what these women need. Anyway, it went horribly wrong, after pushing to get her to go in the first place. That sucked because now I have to work twice as hard to get her to go to another one! You can read more about that below. Mom & I both blogged today because a lot happened, but you should be reading hers first. Oh well, you're mostly through mine now, you might as well continue cause I'm almost done.

Poor little Roxy got sick today and it looked as if there was some blood in her vomit. So, all you prayers', could you please pray for her health too, because I don't think I have it in me to deal with both my girls being sick!!!

'Don't be nice to me!' (2009-02-16 10:07) - CJ

We were looking forward to a fairly easy two-appointment day on Friday, maybe even finishing up early. The drive to Dr. Surgeon's office is about 75 miles round-trip, traffic wasn't too bad and we were there about 15 minutes ahead of time. I got changed into a gown for my mammogram of my left breast (the good one) and sat in the waiting area to be called. When I was taken in for my mammo, who knew 'Dr. Rude's' trainee, 'Radiologist B* & % $' would be doing it! She asked me what was going on and when I told her she said, 'Well, let's get going. You've done enough damage already!' If you've been following this blog, you already know that is the type of comment that reduces me to tears and did.

She finished the mammo and asked me to have a seat while the doc looked at the results. She came back in shortly and said he wanted a couple more pictures. More tears. A few more pictures and wait again. That's when Dr. S. walks in, kisses me on the cheek and asks how I am. Wrong move! We have a thing in our family that when one of us is on the verge of tears and someone offers a hug or caring words, we say, 'don't be nice to me' because we know that kindness will only send us over the edge. And that's exactly what happened! Dr. S. wanted another sonogram of my left breast, the good one.

I'm sure you can imagine what was going through my mind while I waited. I couldn't stop the tears as the sonogram was being done, but the technician was very kind and reassured me throughout the test. More waiting. In the meantime, a woman with a turban wrapped around her head, a sure sign in a cancer center, who was also in the waiting room, came over and sat beside me. She had big tears in her eyes and she said, 'You are making me cry.' She proceeded to tell me that she had just recently completed her chemo and was there to schedule her surgery and for an MRI. She has a husband and three kids, ranging in age from five to 17. She told me how important it is to stay positive, to do what you can do and rest when you need to. She told me about her experience with the chemo and the Neulasta, but in a much less scary way than the 'support' group and with a much more positive outlook. Basically, it is what it is and I've just got to put on my big girl panties and deal with it! Not always as easily done as said!

Dr. S. came into the waiting room, grabbed me by the hand and walked me back to his office. I said, 'Friday the 13th used to be my lucky day. I have a feeling you're about to put an end to that.' Apparently, there are some calcifications in the left breast that just 'don't look right' so he wants to do a biopsy of those as well when I have the port implanted on Tuesday. I told him my fears about the radioactive dye burning like acid, and couldn't they just do it while I'm out. He says it's more like a bee sting but they can't inject radioactive anything in the OR. And then, of course, there's the needle localization for the biopsy. 'While you are positioned for the mammogram, the radiologist will place a needle in the precise spot of the abnormality. Additional mammogram films will be taken to make sure the needle is placed correctly. A thin wire with a small bend at the end will be threaded through the needle to mark the area for biopsy.' Then, of course, once the wire is in place, I will be taken to the OR and will be given a medication to help me relax. TOO LATE! I need the relaxing stuff way before the needle stuff!

So we now head to Admission for my pre-op testing appointment at 1:45. After being told 'you'll be seen shortly' many times, we finally were taken in about 3:15. So much for finishing up on time, let alone early. This one was pretty easy, a review of my medical history, a quick meeting with the anesthesiologist, EKG and blood work, along with a list of instructions for Tuesday.

I'm petrified for Tuesday. I keep telling myself that I've been through lots of junk, I can get through this too, but it doesn't seem to be helping.

Good news, bad news (2009-02-19 10:57) - CJ

Surgery Day, we got to the hospital about 6:40 a.m., got signed in and proceeded to Mammography. Another mammo of my left breast to determine the exact location of the calcifications they wanted to biopsy, Lidocaine to numb the area and a wire inserted to mark the spot for Dr. S. Then six sticks of a needle to insert the dye around the tumor of the right breast to send it to the sentinel node. I have determined that I will no longer listen to the doom and gloom of the 'support' group, as it was nowhere near as bad as they told me it would be! From now on, only POSITIVE support!

From there I was sent to 'suit up' for surgery. They now have matching gowns and socks and the gowns have a little pocket in them to hook up a hose, which sends warm air into the gown! Pretty neat since they keep it like an icebox in there! Assorted docs, residents, nurses and techs came in to do their thing and the one thing that was consistent, from the time I was admitted until the time I was discharged, was that everyone told me I have the BEST doctor! He came in to reassure me once again and to 'bump foreheads' with me like he does with his kids! Hugs and kisses with Beth and Janice and off I went.

I woke up in the recovery room sometime around noon, vaguely remember seeing my daughter and sister and Dr. S. He said the calcifications were fine, but the sentinel node is malignant, totally opposite of what the sonogram and the needle biopsy had shown.

I was given a saltine and a sip of water, a pain pill, then back to dreamland. Several times when I woke, a nurse was applying lots of pressure on the port site and she explained that was because it kept swelling. Dr. S. came in and explained that they were going to take me back to surgery to aspirate a hematoma that was causing the swelling but had to wait until about 3 p.m. because of the saltine I had eaten. Later, the anesthesiologist came in to explain about the tubes they would have to put down my throat since I had eaten that huge saltine (sounds scary but I was out and didn't even know it) and that I would have a bit of a sore throat afterward. More hugs and kisses and off once again. I remember asking the resident if they still play music in the OR. He seemed to get a kick out of that.

The next time I woke up in recovery I have no idea what time it was, but there had been a changing of the guards and I had a new nurse. Dr. S. came in to check on me and I remember him apologizing for the second surgery, but that he wouldn't have been able to sleep that night if he hadn't taken me back in.

Finally, I was released, we got home around 9:30 p.m. and Beth got me settled in. She's such a little worry-wart. Would she be able to hear me if I needed her, would she know what to do, would I fall if I tried to get up, did I have everything I needed. And as a result, she got very little sleep. I, on the other hand, slept like a baby.

Beth was up early on Wednesday to pick up Roxy from the kennel. She hates being in the kennel. The poor little thing won't eat while she's there and just sits and shakes. Beth brought her in to see Grammy in a more 'controlled' manner than the usual jumping and licking! We decided that what we all needed the most was a 'snow day', so we pulled the blinds, turned off the phones and slept all day!

Beth and Jan, in case I didn't tell you, in my groggy state, I love you girls and appreciate your support more than you know!

Update (2009-02-24 10:16) - CJ

I have been having lots of pain in my right breast the past several days. The docs feel that the chemo will help that. They think the pain is being caused because the tumor is growing and the chemo, hopefully, will shrink it. It literally feels like my skin is going to burst...like when the Incredible Hulk used to burst out of his clothes.

Things that make you say 'hmmm'...the other day in the mail, I received a get well card from the cancer center pre-op and OR staff, and on the same day, a bill from 'Dr. Rude' for my appointment on 12/4! The appointment at which his staff told me there would be no charge as they did NOTHING!

Chemo starts 2/26...please keep those prayers coming!! And by the way, for those of you who have asked, Dr. S. describes the sentinel node as the 'keeper of the castle'. If it is clear of cancer, they can be sure the cancer has not invaded the lymph nodes. In my case, of course, that is not the case, so they will have to remove lymph nodes when they do the mastectomy.

You can't judge a book by its cover . . .
(2009-02-25 12:21) - Beth

WOW, what a day we had today! I'm not really going into the technical details, basically because I really don't remember them at this point, as it is only three hours since we've been home from this 15-hour journey. Today mom had three surgeries scheduled. Mom, Janny & I head out for Moffitt at 5:30 am. All of us running on very little sleep and highly stressful situations. Mom's emotions are getting the best of her and the poor little thing is in tears during the easiest part of all, admin. She is so frightened of the pain and rightfully so! After admin, we head to the breast clinic for a mammogram and the insertion of a wire, which will remain so they are able to cut out the correct area for testing (which is allegedly very painful as if they were shooting acid under her skin). This she feared the most. Turns out, this wasn't even close to what she had been told. There was some pain but wasn't bad at all and she begins to relax a little. Although that relaxation could have been generated by the Vicodin and valium she was utilizing to calm her nerves. Off to Pre-Op.

Everyone was so great! They all introduced themselves and it was very calming to know they were going to be with my mother when I was forbidden. I thought we would have some time to just hang out a little before they whisked her off to surgery, but NO, they were waiting for her. Time for her to go. That's not enough time to express to someone who means so much, just how much you love them. There is always a risk when someone goes under the knife that they won't come out of it. 'Don't cry - Don't cry - Don't cry', I continually repeated to myself. I am the strong one. I cannot let them wheel my mother away to a surgery that she is so frightened of and the last thing she sees is me . . . crying. She needs my strength and I will prevail!

Okay, now Janny & I have to find something to do to keep our minds off the situation. I've been trying desperately to NOT worry about things that I cannot change. Humor always works. Our family is particularly funny! Let's make each other laugh. Okay, that works. Let's get some other people involved. This is a surgical waiting room in a cancer clinic. Clearly, everyone here is under an immeasurable amount of stress and could use a laugh. I love to make people laugh. Somehow, when other people laugh, that makes me happy inside. I enjoy seeing others have happy times in the moment. And, sometimes you have to laugh to keep from crying!

Okay, now what? It's always fun to flirt with some hot guys (of course, if you can find any). Turns out, the supervisor for valet is pretty hot. Let's keep an eye on him. Oddly, he must have been doing the same with me. Janny & I decide to go to the cafeteria and see him working and casually give a glance. As we're getting off the elevator in another building, he is walking by at that exact moment. Hmm, can you say 'Hot Stalker'?

Doc S. came to tell us that mom had to go back into surgery because she was swelling at the port site and he was concerned. Oh God, what happened to it going well about an hour ago? He said one of us could go back and see her. Of course, that would be me! She looked so weak and frail. The tears begin to burn my eyes. Keep blinking, that always works. Blink, blink.

I was sent away again as they took her back to surgery. Okay, call the kennel and check on your other girl. She is not eating and has not eaten since I dropped her off on Monday evening at 5 pm. I miss her so much. More tears swelling and Janny's watching. Hmm, good time for a bathroom break. 'Get it together', I told myself in the bathroom.

Anyway, long story short . . . I started this entry three hours after we came home that day, but for some reason, couldn't bring myself to complete it until now. Sorry for the delay. The moral of the story . . . You can't judge a book by its cover because on the outside I appear very tough and can handle anything. However, on the inside, I feel as if I am falling apart, literally and my skin is the only thing holding my body together!

I'm curious as to just how much strength I really do possess before I actually snap. I'm hoping that doesn't happen, but you hear about it all the time. Anyway, I am rambling now so I shall end here . . .

project 'I am Beautiful' **(2009-02-25 17:00) - Beth**

Today was a VERY productive, good day for us here. I had mentioned in one of my previous posts about a new vision that we are working on and I feel ready to announce it to you all. I have been very excited about this vision and can't wait to get started with the 'planning' stage, which is right after the 'secure funding' stage!

Today I had lunch with a very dear friend of mine (which was a pleasure in itself as we haven't had much time together lately, thanks TG!) and this guy is a good one to know for his wealth of knowledge, particularly about this type of thing. We discussed my vision and he thinks it is a really solid idea. He is going to reach out to some of his resources and see if he can hook me up with some folks who might be able to assist me in getting this project off the ground. I don't think I've ever been more excited about a project in my life!

On a lighter note... (2009-02-26 17:10) - CJ

I had my first chemo treatment this morning and as I write this (about 5 p.m.), I can honestly say the only thing I am feeling is very sleepy. I will write more about this tomorrow when I can hopefully say, 'NO side effects'.

But for today, I wanted to try something different. I figure that when y'all read the blog, you're either bored to tears by all my medical details or crying tears of emotions reading my precious daughter's feelings as we go through this. Well, today we're going to LAUGH!!!

You've all read about how Beth and I have implemented The Memory Vase and how it is one of our favorite daily routines. It never fails to bring laughter to us each day when we each read a 'remember when' card. Here I would like to share with you, some memories I have about some of you who are reading this.

Joey P...RW as kids, I was chasing you through the house for some reason. We got to the living room where you went down on your knees and I went ass-over-tin cups over top of you?!!

Bobby...RW you woke up one morning, after listening to Phyllis Hyman sing 'Gonna' Make Changes' on auto play all night, and said, 'If that bitch makes one more change...'?!!

Heidi...RW we were at a picnic at Joey P.'s, you took a bite of corn on the cob, went to say something and a kernel of corn went flying...from your mouth right into Janice's mouth?!!

Lauren...RW I used to watch you while your mom worked and we made up silly games to play in the pool?!!

Bob T...RW, in response to someone questioning your size in pants, you said, 'Well, I wear 34's, but 36's feel so good that I buy 38's'?!!

Hayley...RW Bethie and I met you and your parents at Disney and you put on a dancing show in front of the HUGE crowd that had gathered to watch and clap for you?!!

Joe G...RW I said it was hot in your house and you said, 'Take off your shirt and stand under the fan'?!!

Lisa...RW I gave you a back-to-school perm and put the neutralizer on BEFORE the curl solution? (Sorry about that!!)

Michelle...RW we used to go to the races and you brought not only hot chocolate but also marshmallows?!!

Andy...RW I used to watch you when your mom worked and you always wanted to know if we could go to Tom's for lunch (meaning Jerry's)?!!

John...RW as young teenagers we couldn't wait to go to picnics or parties where we could do our cha-cha?!! (People clapped for us too, Hayley!!)

Jan...RW we spent hours upon hours at my house doing the '...And We Know Funny' book?!! Too bad WE didn't have any fun!!

Cyndi...RW you and your mom and Beth and I went to Safety Harbor for a girls' spa weekend?

Ashley...RW, at age 13, you said to me, 'Aunt Carol, don't you think I'm getting a little old to be called 'munchkin'?!! (That's when I changed it to Missy!!)

Cindra Lee...RW you came into our family and we told you that if you and John ever broke up, you stay, he goes?!!

Mike P....RW all of us 'grands' used to play 'Mother, May I' in Baba's yard on Easter and Mothers' Day?!!

Tom...RW you, Lynn, Jeff, Beth and I went to the Vinoy to have cocktails after the Main Sail and you got trrrrrashed?!!

Rick...RW you gave me the nickname 'Wandella, the Wonderful Waitress', which was quickly shortened to 'Wan'?!!

I could go on for days...really...but y'all get the idea. Sometimes ya' just gotta' laugh!!

> Anonymous (2009-02-26 19:01:00)
> Carol Laughter is the best medicine. I was watching Joel Osteen the other day and he said it is a scientific fact that laughter produces something in your

body that can cause your body to heal itself EVEN CANCER. I do remember that incident you mentioned and it made me laugh reading it. I hope and pray you have no side effects. I'M PRAYING FOR YOU AND YOUR POSSE.
Love ya joeyp

Anonymous (2009-02-27 06:23:00)
Carol,
RW... you were "putting your affairs in order"? I am so proud of how far you've come and will help in any way I can to keep you going farther.
MONDAY - WE WALK!
By the way, writing "The Book" is one of my happiest memories. I love you!!!
James

Anonymous (2009-03-02 21:06:00)
Yea and I do not remember ever winning at Mother May I. It seems as though the fix was always on. I would get real close and then whack, back to the start. We had loads of fun at Bubba's. Her beef noodle soup with the meat dipped in horseradish (kids eating horseradish, no wonder I have been getting heartburn since I was 18). We were dirt poor and didn't know it or care. We were family enjoying being with family. It is strange (and a little sad) that I really do not remember the things that you do until you share them with me. Just as you did when I visited last April. I can't wait to visit again. I hope to be down in April but we will see (the economy has put a crunch on firm travel but I may still get to come down). I will let you know for sure. So, start banging the brain of yours for all the old memories. I need to remember those times, our times, and I need your help. They are so good to laugh about with you and Beth. And, you know, we will laugh - - guaranteed. Love you both - - Mike

Anonymous (2009-03-08 15:33:00)
CiCi, you're absolutely right, I did laugh out loud, throughout the entire blog! It's funny, I don't think I'd mind so much being "Munchkin" anymore. You can call me whatever you want,... even "Richard". :)
I want to tell you how proud I am of you for coming as far as you have. I really admire your courage. After reading Beth's, it took me a while to come back but I'm finishing it today. It's awesome that both of you are able to express yourselves through this blog and thank you for sharing it with us.
I love you, Ashley

Anonymous (2009-03-16 21:00:00)
Cici, I do remember making up silly games! And all the little tricks I used to show you that I could do in the pool, (that now I look back on, are even

more silly!) I've been reading these blogs every now and then, when I see mommy's on, and it always makes me sad. But hearing that everything's okay makes me feel better. It's probably a little weird to hear this from a little teenager, but I'm proud of you too! I love you, Lauren

2009 March

Chemo Cocktail (2009-03-03 09:37) - CJ

Many years ago someone told me, 'you can't laugh your way through life'. My response was, 'Sometimes that's the ONLY way you can get through it'. I was proven right by the many comments, emails, phone calls and cards we got in response to 'On a lighter note.' I am so glad you all enjoyed the humor in it! Chemotherapy: a type of cancer treatment that uses drugs to destroy cancer cells.

We got to the doc's office for my appointment and chemo treatment. Vitals were taken and blood work drawn to make sure everything was okay to begin the chemo. Dr. O. came in to briefly explain the plan, answered our questions and handed me off to a 'mean' nurse, telling her I was his wife's best friend from Texas (because we have the same name!) (Pay attention, this is relevant later on in the story!)

The chemo room is circled with lounge chairs with IV contraptions on each side. Missy, who was anything but mean, saw that I was on the verge of tears and said she was taking us back to a private room. We went into a room with enough chairs for my 'posse', the standard lounge chair and IV contraptions and a tv. She chatted with us, mostly; I'm sure, to put my mind at ease, while she was getting things 'ready'.

The chemo is administered via the port and this was the first time it would be used, so I was a little nervous. Missy sprayed some kind of freezing spray on it to numb it up and began to hook up the needle. She had to do a little wiggling and it took some time, but I couldn't feel anything because it was numb. Finally, she scores and we begin the treatment.

I got five small bags first, one at a time. These are various drugs to calm me down and help fight nausea. The two chemo drugs that I am receiving during this cycle are Cytoxan and Adriamycin. These ones take about 30–40 minutes, but in all honesty, I actually dozed off. Of course, I'm sure the 'calm me down' drugs were responsible for that!

Every time a bag would empty, the machine would beep and someone would come in to change it, so I got to meet and interact with several nurses. These women are wonderful! Some of them have had a personal experience with cancer and all of them are kind and caring. And talk about dedication, they are even there on weekends and holidays for people who need IV fluids or any other type of help. And Missy is quite funny, as are we! The girls and I had quite a conversation with her concerning 'needles'. We'll just leave it at that!! As we were preparing to leave, Missy told me that I had done fine and, after all, I had a big advantage being the best friend of my doc's wife. I told her that really wasn't true and she has now made it her personal mission to get revenge! I'm afraid Dr. O. is in for some payback!!

All done. I did sleep a good bit that day but felt fine. The next day we go back for the Neulasta shot. The chemo, in its attempt to kill the cancer cells, also, unfortunately, kills some of the good cells, so the Neulasta encourages white cell growth. The problem is, it can also produce flu-like symptoms and bone pain. I was told to take Advil every 4-6 hours, along with my anti-nausea meds.

I felt pretty good until Saturday when I began to have some bone pain, although no worse than those periodic ones we all get, the 'growing pain' kind. The bone pain subsided after a while and on Saturday evening I had a pounding headache and was achy and weepy. I know weepy isn't a flu-like symptom, it's a 'poor me, cancer sucks and I hate this' symptom. Sunday and Monday were pretty much the same but I am feeling a little more human today; hopefully, it will last more than a few hours, for poor Beth's sake!

I am very pleased that I wasn't nauseous. I really hate to throw up. I always said no one would ever have to worry about my being bulimic. But Dr. O. had told me several times that not everyone gets sick and I made up my mind that I would be one of those people who don't.

I go back on Thursday to have blood work done to make sure that my counts are all good, no infections, in preparation for the next chemo treatment the following Thursday.

I have lost a few pounds, but that's not a bad thing since I had actually gained about fifteen pounds just in the two months since I told my family about the cancer! And believe it or not, there's no such thing as 'chemo-skinny' anymore. Now they tell you to expect to GAIN 20-30 pounds! Talk about adding insult to injury!! Now, however, not a lot of food tastes good to me, a side effect, plus the roof of my mouth is sore, another side effect. I have not had a chocolate coke in about four weeks and there's a bag of chocolate covered pretzels on the counter that have been there since last Thursday. For those of you who know me...WHAT???!!!

What Cancer Cannot Do (2009-03-06 16:41) - CJ

I really thought I breezed through my first chemo treatment. I took my 'don't throw up' medicine for the first three days as prescribed and was so pleasantly surprised that I really didn't get nauseous until Tuesday. I was so sick, achy and tired that all I could do was sit and cry. Of course, the aching is from the Neulasta and apparently, there is no expiration date on nausea (memories of pregnancy!) However, today is the first time I have actually thrown up. I am back on the antiemetic to try to control it. I try to eat something light and somewhat bland in between bouts, but nothing much really sounds good to me these days. I am trying to be somewhat active, but honestly, after about a half-hour, have to rest. Beth and I went to the grocery store the other day and 50 minutes did me in!

Another side effect of the chemotherapy is constipation, so now we have to add Milk of Magnesia to the mix. Yum.

Yesterday I went for my blood work. They have to monitor my white blood cells, red blood cells, and platelets in preparation for my next chemo treatment in a week. My white count had gone from 13.1 last week to 1.5 this week. This, apparently, is normal because the Neulasta takes two weeks to actually start building the white count back up. It has to be greater than 3 in order to get the next chemo and they tell me that it will be.

Because I cry at the drop of a hat these days, Dr. O. has put me on Paxil for depression and I have been scheduled a (hopefully) routine appointment with Dr. Shrink. The general consensus at this point seems to be that, since I kept this to myself for almost two years, it's 'in my face' now and there is no more denying, so it's kind of like I'm just finding out about it myself. Throw in the fact that I hate to burden Beth any more than I already am, so yeah, I guess I do need to talk with someone impartial.

Janice came over last night to spend some quality time, not in a doctor's office or hospital! She brought me a book called, 'What Cancer Cannot Do'. For those of you who are not familiar:

Cancer is so limited

It cannot cripple Love
It cannot shatter Hope
It cannot corrode Faith
It cannot kill Friendship
It cannot suppress Memories
It cannot silence Courage
It cannot invade the Soul
It cannot steal eternal Life
It cannot conquer the Spirit

It is a book of stories of hope and encouragement and James, I appreciate it, and you, more than you know. The three of us and little Roxy just hung out and laughed our faces off. We all needed it SO much. THANK YOU, GIRLS!!

Oprah called . . . (2009-03-06 21:06) - Beth

Wow, sorry it's been so long since I've blogged, but you wouldn't believe what's been happening. Ever since I posted the blog *project: 'I am Beautiful'*, it's been crazy around here! Apparently, the word got out about the project and I've had to hire a personal assistant to field calls for me. Calls from the press, television networks, even Oprah herself wanting to interview me and write the forward for my book. Then I get a call from Sheryl Crow. Being a breast cancer survivor herself, she loved what I was doing and begged to be included in the book. She's flying me to Greece where she is doing some shows and I will hold her photo shoot there. Not to mention, I've already obtained pre-orders of the book in excess of 100,000, which has surpassed my expected goal of raising $5 million for funding for non-medical expenses (e.g., mortgage, utilities, groceries, etc.) for women fighting breast cancer, which will allow these women to concentrate solely on healing both physically and emotionally.

Okay, so none of this has happened yet, but they say you have to visualize it to make it happen. However, some news in a positive direction, a friend of mine turned me on to a plastic surgeon that thinks the project is very 'important' as he does a lot of reconstructive surgery for breast cancer survivors. I am meeting with him on Wednesday to discuss the project in more detail. He actually thanked my friend for mentioning it to him. This really just tickles me pink. I NEED to do this project! If I could possibly be selfish for a moment, although I'm not sure you could really use the word 'selfish' when discussing any part of this project, I can't wait for the experience it is going to bring me. Meeting all the courageous women I'm about to meet, I can only imagine, will be so empowering to me. What an impact it will leave knowing these women are going from surviving to thriving. So, wish me luck!

More 'angels' (2009-03-08 11:57) - CJ

For those of you who are disappointed when we don't blog every day (Joey P.!!), here's another.

Beth and I are so blessed to have so many wonderful family members and friends! Some of these people have been our friends for over half of my life (that's a really long time!) and for most of Beth's. We are also blessed to have met so many new people who will, undoubtedly, become friends.

More thank-yous!

Michelle and Dennis, thank you so much for the great card and for the check! And Dennis, I want you to know that the mirror you made me for Christmas about a mazillion years ago is still used every single day!

Jane, from Dr. O.'s office, thank you so much for the book you gave me the other day. It is very inspirational and I am enjoying and learning from it! Thank you also for all your suggestions regarding resources, as well as our blog.

Joe G, thank you so much for taking my 'posse' out for the evening and making them laugh! Believe me, they need it after hanging around with me for a couple hours!! I know you all had a good time and the girls really needed it! In addition, thank you so much for the washer! (Ours went south the other day because, of course, when it rains, it pours and Joe and Jan went out and got us another, brought it over and installed it!! Not only that, but Joe has insisted on doing our lawn until we get back on our feet!) Thank you for that, too, Big Daddy, you're the greatest!

John, thank you so much for the great conversation we had yesterday. Even though you are going through a ton of your own junk, you had the time to boost me up when I needed it! (And by the way, I am so glad that you have finally had some good news!!)

Rich, thank you so much for the check, it will certainly come in handy! Thanks also for the articles and for your prayers!

Joey P, thank you so much for reading the blog every day! Thank you for our phone call this morning (3 hours!). I always love talking with you and I can't wait till you get down here so we can spend some quality time together. And I am 'keeping a tally' for you!!

Andy & Heidi, thank you so much for the beautiful card and all your prayers! We can't wait to see you guys and those little rug rats!

I know a lot of you have sent emails because you are having trouble posting comments on the blog. We appreciate and enjoy your emails and want you to know that Beth is working on a solution for the blog comments, as we want to hear your thoughts.

We love and appreciate you all more than you know!!

Adding Comments (2009-03-08 16:16) - Beth

It has been brought to my attention that there are some issues when adding comments. Sometimes they go through and sometimes they don't. We really love hearing your comments and, although, we are getting comments via email . . . we'd really like them to be posted to the blog itself. I would recommend that if you are attempting to post a comment directly to the blog, type it in Word or Notepad first, that way if it doesn't post, you won't lose all the words and feelings you just spent the time writing. That has happened in several situations.

If you are having difficulty posting comments, please email me your comments and indicate you want them posted (I don't want to post anything meant for a personal email) and I will post them on the blog. Oh, also indicate the title of the blog you want the comment posted to. Okay, so you all want us to update the blog every day . . . we also would like to see your comments every day!

Thanks for all of your support and the comments that have been added. Reading those encourages us to blog more.

Love to all!

Girls' Night Out (2009-03-09 22:21) - CJ

Beth, Janice and I went to a support group meeting tonight called 'Look Good, Feel Better'. This was much different from the last and way more fun! There were about ten of us who are going through different stages of treatment and several friends and family. They gave us kits filled with just about every type of makeup a girl could wish for! And it was all name brand too, not the five & dime stuff! (I know, probably most of you don't even know what a five & dime is.)

Karen, the 'wigist' (who knew THAT was a word?) explained how important it is to avoid infection when going through chemo because your resistance is so low. She showed us how to apply makeup to compensate for the loss of eyebrows and eyelashes and I was in 'full makeup' for the first time in years! Of course, my problem is that I can't see to apply the darn stuff! The things I have always liked best about myself were my boobs and my eyes...and three out of four have let me down!

She also had bags of scarfs, hats, turbans, and wigs donated by the Cancer Society and it was fun going through them and picking out different things. I got a couple scarves and a straw hat to wear if I have to be in the sun, although they frown on that. Pretty tough for a former diehard sun-worshipper!

Anyhow, the girls said I looked so pretty we should go out, so we went for a sandwich. Home by 9:15...we're such lightweights!

This is actually the first day in quite a while that I have felt human. I go for my next chemo treatment on Thursday and I will continue to have positive thoughts regarding that!

Miss Hayley (2009-03-09 22:49) - CJ

This is a little note for Miss Hayley...I apologize for spelling your name wrong. Of course, I know how to spell it, and when I was typing it didn't look quite right, but I figured 'sure, it's right'. And then I asked Bethie and she told me I was W-R-O-N-G, so I fixed it...did you notice? Aunt Cici is age-challenged, but I promise never to misspell it again! I love you, sweetie!

She's so cute! (2009-03-10 00:01) - Beth

Watching mom at the 'Look Good - Feel Better' group tonight, she is so stinkin' cute! Tonight was much like the conversation I had with my mom last night about little Roxy. I told her that every time I look at her I have to smile or even giggle because Roxy is just so darned cute. Those are the same feelings I had about mom tonight. I think she really got into this support group. Normally shy, she didn't hesitate to speak up and ask questions or answer them. I was very proud of her! And then watching her apply the makeup and crack jokes about not being able to see what she is doing or laughing about how uneven she drew her eyebrows in, that was really great for me. I can't tell you how much it means to me that she is feeling good today!! I even got a commitment from her for tomorrow. We have to go see Dr. Shrink tomorrow and I had her promise that upon returning home, we would take Roxy to 'Roxy Park'. She does think she owns it and will chase all the big birds away and she struts her stuff around that park, as does my mom!

Mom's been craving a margarita since she's 'looked good and felt better,' we decided to go get her one. One is, after all, all she can handle! It's so funny because my mom is not a drinker. Don't get me wrong, I'm not saying she's NEVER been a drinker. I remember one time asking as a child, 'Why's my mom behind the couch?' Her laughing and responding, 'I'm okay.' And you have to know her laugh to appreciate this. She has one of those contagious laughs that when she laughs, EVERYONE laughs!

So, during her first appointments, they've asked her if she's a drinker and ever since she's said 'No, I'm not a drinker', she drinks more. It reminds me of the story of my Great-Grandmother never smoking a day in her life until the day she found out she had cancer. It makes me chuckle to see mom intoxicated, especially from one drink.

We were teasing her during her first chemo treatment about the liquid they pumped into her that calmed her nerves. They call that a 'glass of red wine' and that is the effect it had on her. She was cute then, too.

Okay, so here's something a little strange that you probably don't know about us unless you're family. Do you remember 'Ghost' the movie? Well, we decided that we didn't want to be in the position of not knowing if someone was coming back for real or not. So, we came up with initials to a long saying that only the two of us know and whenever one of us passes, we'll know whether or not it is really the other coming back. We say the initials in front of others, but nobody knows the full wording. We did it before and Janny figured it out so we were forced to change it. This isn't something we've come up with since cancer. We've been doing this since 'Ghost' came out.

I am aware that my mom is fighting this, all for me. She doesn't want to leave me alone. I don't think she could know how much I love her, although, she says the same to me. She is my best friend in the whole world!! And I can't possibly imagine life without her. I am so lucky that we have the relationship that we do. I can't begin to explain what it feels like to think about losing such an important person in your life. I can only hope and pray that she makes it for another 15 to 20 years or longer, but especially until she sees what it was all for. We believe that all things happen for a reason and if the reason is to aid women dealing with breast cancer through the book that I hope to create, then it was all for a reason. But she can't leave me! I don't think I can make it without her.

> Anonymous (2009-03-12 19:25:00)
> Beth, It is so awesome to see that you love your mom so much and 'will' do anything for her. I am sure that she thinks that having you as her daughter and the relationship that you two have is worth it all. I know that I would and do feel the same about my mom and my prayer is that Hayley will feel that

way about me someday. I love you both and keep praying for you and CiCi. Hope to see you soon. Heidi

Mom thanked us today . . . (2009-03-12 20:20) - Beth

We went for mom's second chemo treatment today and she met with Dr. O. He was very pleased with her responses upon asking her how the first treatment turned out. She was nauseous some after the second week, but only vomited once. He was also pleased when he looked at her breast. He made the same comment I did when I looked at this morning before we left the house. Dr. O and I both thought the color looked better and it didn't look so tight. You have to understand this lump is, literally, the size of a baseball. You know when women are pregnant and their bellies stretch to accommodate the baby, which is what her breast did to accommodate the size of this lump. It made her right breast noticeably larger than her left. Since it didn't look as tight, is a good indication that the chemo is doing what it is supposed to be doing. He is certain that it is going to continue to decrease the size of this cancer.

Anyway, we got her situated and she began her many 'bags-o-chemo'. Mom thanked Janny and me for convincing her to get treatment because it really wasn't as bad as she had herself convinced it would be. And we thanked her for deciding to go through with treatment.

This poor little adorable older woman was sitting two seats from my mother and they were poking her over and over with a needle trying to make it into her vein, but her veins kept giving out and collapsing. Poor thing was all alone and she continued to shake her feet as they tortured her with that needle. Particularly weepy today, I couldn't help but go over and hold her hand. I thought I would burst into tears when I took her hand in mine and told her, 'Honey, squeeze my hand. You shouldn't be going through this alone!'

When my new-found friend was all situated and mom was getting drowsy from the Benadryl, Janny asked if I wanted to go for a walk. She was my rock today and I want to thank you, Janny, for being just that! During our walk, I asked her for a favor. Yesterday, I asked mom if she was going to have her head shaved and she said she was just going to cut it herself real short and might need my help for the back. I've been hesitating to post this, but if I am to be honest, then I have to be just that. Although I know that mom losing her hair is imminent, that is the hardest for me to deal with. And I know it is for my mom too and I want to be strong for her. Anyway, I asked Janny if she could do this for me. She told me to just say the word, wait now that I think about it, was she wanting to hear . . . please? You know I always have to throw some humor in there. Nevertheless, Janny remained and helped me through the day with winks, smiles, and humor!

We stop at the store to get prescriptions filled and continued home; Six hours later, exhausted and really needing a good cry.

I never had that 'good cry' but I did have several hours of much-needed sleep. This really is exhausting!! But we do what we have to because . . . we love each other!!!

> Anonymous (2009-03-13 08:29:00)
> When I read this, it makes all the things I am going through seem so insignificant and petty compared to what you are going through.
> Carol, you are such an inspiration to me. You have to be one of the strongest people I know. You have taken this on full force and are refusing to give up. There has been sometimes lately that I have thrown up my hands and said, "I am done, I can't do this anymore." Then I read your blog and you instill me with the attitude that nothing is going to put me down for the count. You have given me the attitude that nothing can keep you down if you don't want it to. For this, I thank you with all my heart.
> To the "posse". You guys are amazing. You do things that most people

wouldn't think to do in helping someone and it comes naturally to you both. I have found that with support from the people you love, that things sometimes don't look as bad as you think and you can accomplish so much more.

Anyway, keep the blog going, I see a best seller when everything is done.

I say my novena to St Jude every day and He knows your names, as well as he, knows mine now. I love you both and will be waiting for the next post.

Love you, John

PS Carol, thanks for the phone conversation the other day. It let me get some things said that I haven't told anyone before. How great is that, that someone going through what you are going through takes the time to help someone else? You are the best...

More issues than Playboy! (2009-03-13 23:59) - CJ

It's been several days since I've posted, so I'll start with Dr. Shrink. I went to see her on Tuesday and really like her. She doesn't think I need 'fixed', but that with so much going on in the past year, losing a brother and my mom, the financial situation, the cancer and keeping it a secret for so long. It's a lot on my plate. And she has vowed to help me work through it. What a relief!

Thursday I went to see Dr. O and he thinks the tumor is shrinking, good news! I also had my chemo and so far, so good. My little Florence Nightingale felt so much compassion for the woman who was getting poked and prodded while they tried to find a vein; she went over and held her hand, got her water and just comforted her, in general. Then she turned into Julie, the cruise director, and talked with another woman about her scarf and where she got it.

All the nurses are so kind. You would think it would be a depressing place to work, but they feel that they are helping to heal people and they are always so cheerful, which does wonders for morale! On chemo day, I pretty much sleep all day because of all the drugs they give me. Works for me. I was able to eat a little and with the Compazine, had no nausea.

Friday I went for my Neulasta shot and am adamantly taking Advil to help ward off the bone pain. It makes me very tired and I had a 'little' five-hour nap!

I am now ready to admit that I am glad I was able to be persuaded by Beth, Janice and all my family and friends to have treatment. It really is not as bad as I thought it would be. Don't get me wrong, it's no walk in the park and I still have my bad days, but I also have good days, and after all, I'm still here with my precious daughter.

Beth is having a hard time with the 'hair' thing. It's starting to fall out and I will have to make a decision soon whether to shave it or just watch it fall out daily. I'm having a hard time with it as well because I hate my ears! There have been several suggestions for that dilemma. Joey P. suggested cutting them off, but then what would hold up my glasses? I think we've decided on Gorilla Glue!!

Jan, I want to thank you for being Beth's rock on Thursday. She always tries to be so strong for me and forgets sometimes, that she needs a rock.

Thanks so much for all the comments we are getting. We welcome them all!

Chemo Kicker (2009-03-16 13:45) - Beth

It's happening. We knew it was inevitable. Mom's hair is no longer shedding, but coming out in clumps now and it's just a frightening experience. It is very difficult for my mom to deal with. She said it's almost worse than losing her breast; however, I think her thoughts on that will change once she's had time to deal with the hair loss. She did cut it short this morning to try to get used to this new look. I actually thought it looked pretty cute, but she didn't (with the whole 'ear' thing). It actually took longer than they initially told us.

They said it would fall out within 10-14 days and it's been 18 days since her first chemo treatment.

I told my mom that I would shave my head if that would make her feel better. She said she would never ask me to do that and I told her that she didn't 'ask' me. Then she said not to because she doesn't plan on going out without a wig or scarf. I might still do it. One can never tell what actions might come from me!!

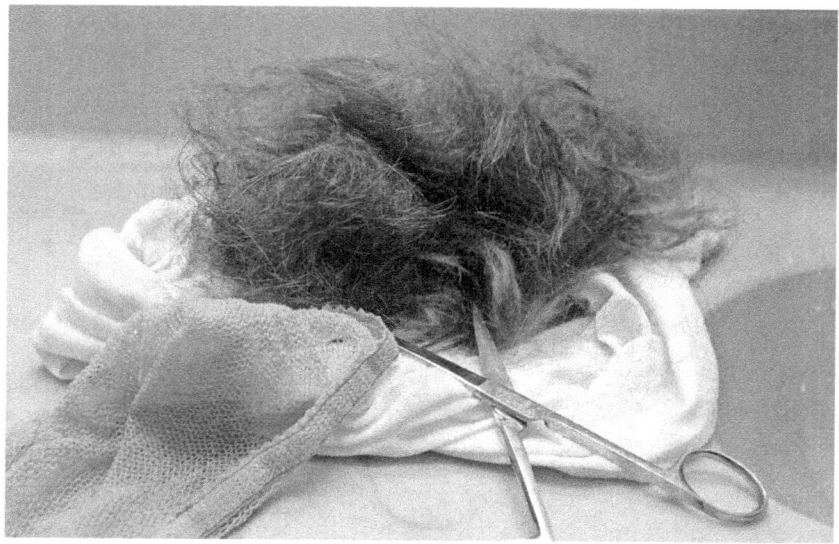

You know, as silly as it sounds, our hair makes a statement about us as women. All of our lives we are trained not to leave the house until our make-up and hair are just perfect. We make an effort to look and feel as beautiful as we possibly can. Then cancer strikes . . . leaving these women hairless & breastless. These are the two most important differences that define a woman.

On a lighter note, I've trained my mother well. I've taught her that the success in gift-giving comes when you can create tears from others. She loves the team that has gathered around to heal her so much that she took gifts on Friday.

She took great pride in picking several stained glass hearts that she had previously made for each department: front desk, chemo nurses, blood work nurses, Dr. O, the foundation directors (who managed to find funding to help us with our mortgage payment this month . . . 'God bless them!!') and one special little girl. Mom's so cute, she even handpicked the wrapping color to correspond to the department (i.e., red for blood work nurses, etc.).

It was a success as she managed to get some tears of gratitude flowing. Particularly with one chemo nurse, who during our first visit explained that her daughter was diagnosed with an odd type of brain cancer. This little girl made such an impact on my mother as she thought, 'If this little girl can fight cancer, surely I can do it too!' My mom gave her a heart to give to her daughter because she inspired my mother to keep fighting. It turns out, that particular day was Sarah's second anniversary of being cancer free. Talk about perfect timing! She is four years old now, has a twin brother and is doing great. God bless her for helping my mother fight this battle!!

God bless the entire team!!

Capturing the facts . . . (2009-03-17 00:39) - Beth

You know one of my favorite things to do is pick up my camera and capture the facts. I particularly like to shoot things out of the norm. Not what a person's eye would normally see, but perhaps a close-up of something that you really have to study to figure out what the big picture is. I love to shoot things that, I guess, make you go hmmm. I remember shooting a fruit stand in New York. The shot turned out to be a close-up of some bananas and other fruit. A gay friend of mine 'got it' right away and thought it was an award winner. My God-daughter, on the other hand, said 'Bethie, it's fruit!'

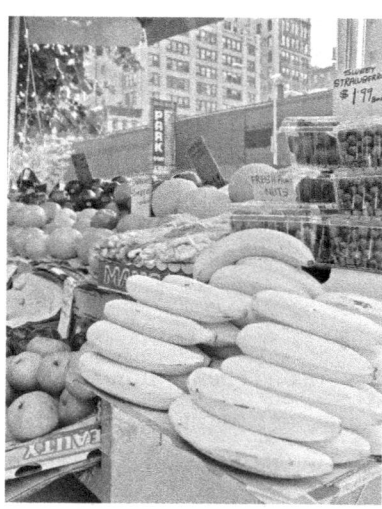

While talking with my Australian friend (and fellow photographer) the other day, he said I should be posting more pictures on the blog. When I began to think about how much I love being behind the camera, I wondered why I wasn't doing what I know makes me happy when I have so much stress in my life right now. I would think that would make me feel better! I've come to a conclusion, it's because we are all masochists. How many of us need to exercise and know that when we do . . . we feel better? Yet, something keeps us from doing the very things that make us feel better. What the hell is wrong with us? What the hell is wrong with me??

Okay, so I'm determined to pick up the camera again. I think for my own sake, I need to document photographically, what life is like around here. Don't worry, I don't shoot overly morbid, but I do think it's important to capture the facts. I want you all to push me on this. Of course, I will share my images with those of you that care to see them.

I thought I wanted to be a photographic journalist for a while before it dawned on me that I was a sap and would be constantly crying hearing other people's stories.

But . . . this is our story! I feel I would be letting us and others down if I didn't start capturing the facts.

But Dude, that's not even my church! (2009-03-18 01:00) - CJ

Joey P. is very spiritual and a real inspiration to the rest of the family. A couple weeks ago in one of our 'short' (three hour) phone conversations, he told me this story. The church that Andy and Heidi go to is building a new Life Center and they are looking for volunteers to help with all phases of the construction. Joey P. was talking with God one night and received a message that God wanted him to help with the building. Joey P.'s response was, 'But Dude, that's not even my church'. Again God told him that He wanted him to help with the building and again, Joey P. responded, 'Dude, that's not my church'. Apparently, God was pretty persistent and Joey P. decided to volunteer!

The next morning on their way to work, (they're drywallers), Andy told his dad that he had received a message from God that he wanted Andy to help with the Life Center. When Joey P. told Andy he had received the same message, Andy's response was, 'But Dude, that's not even your church'. (Like father, like son!)

Needless to say, they volunteered to work on Andy's church Life Center. Joey P., always the negotiator, told God that all the blessings he would receive from it, he wanted to be passed on to me, 100 %.

He told me, that just out of curiosity; he wanted me to keep a tally of each blessing I received, even if it was someone being compassionate at a doctor's appointment. I did as he asked and in seven days, we received eight blessings! This is the email I sent him:

Dear Joe...

Washer from Joe and Jan. Joe's offer to do our lawn free till we get back on our feet. A card from mom (Mary Lou). Food stamp card for $367 a month (It actually came at 10:44 a.m. on the day I opened the email that said I was going to have a blessing at 11:00 a.m.)

I found out Medicaid paid my $3300 emergency room bill (but it wasn't supposed to be in effect until January and I found out about it at 11:05 a.m. the day the email said I would get a blessing at 11:09). Our local Oncology Foundation paid March's mortgage and will pay the electric and water bills and Beth's car insurance.

A great voicemail from Michelle and Dennis saying how heartfelt and honest the blog is and how much they love us and are thinking of us.

Another card from mom along with her church bulletin asking for daily prayers for her daughter-in-law. So do you think you've been rewarded enough for working on a church that isn't even yours?!!!

Thank you so much for the blessings!!!

I love you!

me xox

> anonymous (2009-03-18 01:29:00)
> Carol, That is so awesome to hear all of the blessings that you've been receiving, as well as how well you are doing with the chemo. Make sure you let people know how good GOD is and how he keeps his promises to all who trust him for all their needs. Keep on keeping track of these blessings, because I'm sure there are more coming. Remember you can't out give God. Thanks so much for keeping such a positive attitude through this ordeal; it makes my heart feel good knowing that you aren't giving up. By the way, another blessing

is the posse that you have surrounding you, (Beth, Janice, and your many guardian angels that you can't physically see, but God has sent to hold you up when you think you can't take anymore). I'm still being blessed every day by your blog, thanks for keeping it updated. By the way, Mom and Dad would be very proud of you for your strength and courage. I love you joeyp

No more bad hair days! (2009-03-20 18:24) - CJ

There are some pros to being bald. It certainly cuts down on 'getting ready' time (I can probably beat Joey now!), no hair products to buy, your look depends on your mood each day now, not your hair!

This week has been particularly bad, continually nauseous and unbelievably tired. And not debilitating but just as annoying, I get this shaky, raspy, 'Katherine Hepburn' voice when I have the chemo. In addition, my hair started falling out on Monday, and yes, it IS traumatic. If you just touch your head, you come away with a handful of hair. I cut it short but it didn't look much better. It makes your scalp so tender that even the shower hurts it.

I went for a 10-minute blood work appointment on Thursday and because of nausea and fatigue, they decided to give me additional IV fluids. Two hours later, we headed for the wig shop.

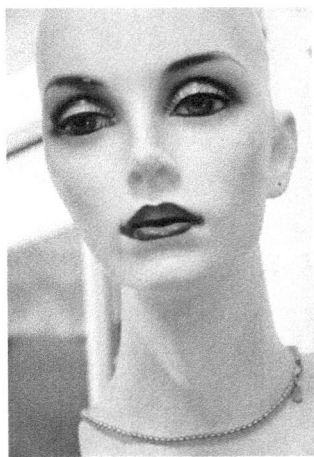

The women there are so kind and fun, as well as knowledgeable. Three of the five are cancer survivors, so they are all very compassionate. I knew they did buzz cuts at this shop, so I opted for that. For about two hours, I tried on wigs and scarves, finally deciding on two very different looks, a short, blond bob, a longer, spikier, frosted, textured cut and a really cute scarf with several different looks. All of this ($496) was paid for through a breast cancer fund that we had heard about, thankfully. Actually, I was the last client to be able to access this resource because the sad thing is that the fund has not been renewed for next year. It's so important to feel good through the treatment of this disease. This is one of the things Beth wants to help with through *project: 'I Am Beautiful'*.

I wore the short one home and Roxy jumped around barking at me! It's so comical! She does that every time I put on a wig or head covering as if to say, 'You smell like Grammy, you taste like Grammy, but you don't LOOK like Grammy!'

I tried to take a little nap with no luck, so Beth and I had a bite to eat and watched a little tv and I was able to get a decent night's sleep with a little help from my 'friends'. I'm counting on feeling much better today, as my chores are backing up! And we haven't found a fund yet that pays for maids!! ;)

Post-op Appointment (2009-03-24 22:39) - Beth

We made the journey back to see Dr. S. in Tampa today for mom's post-op appointment. Man, it was freezing in there!! Dr. S. was so happy to see my mom & the progress that the chemo has made. I don't know if it's because she reminds him of his own mother or just because she was so scared of any kind of treatment at all or maybe just because she is so stinkin' sweet, but I do think he really feels a special bond with her. He continually apologized for having to take her back into surgery during her first surgeries, but he said he would not have been able to sleep that night with the port ballooning up like it was had he not. He didn't want us to be on the interstate heading back to St. Pete and something happen. Yeah . . . neither would we!! So, mom took a special gift for him . . . an angel that she made in stained glass because 'he was her angel'. Then, she 'forgot' to tell him after he opened it that she made it and the whole angel story. Both of those were the best part of the gift. He was very much appreciative, hugged her and told her he loved her.

All in all, this was a very good trip. And there wasn't much traffic to speak of either, so that's the time to go. Oh, I almost forgot . . . he loved our new mission *project: 'I am Beautiful'*!

He said he would pass it on to the support groups because he believes that all women should be made to feel like women and he really recognized the importance in this area.

On our way home, we had to stop and drop off our donations for the fashion show/silent auction that is coming in May that will benefit the foundation. Mom donated a piece of stained glass and me, a framed photo. It feels really good to give back to those that have helped you, but I want to pay it forward also. That is why I am so passionate about *project: 'I am Beautiful*!! And I also know that when this project takes off the way I have visualized, and then I will be able to benefit this foundation even more.

> Anonymous (2009-03-26 10:38:00)
> Just checking in and getting the new update. I am glad you had a 'good day with the Dr.' We are so happy that you have such a wonderful Dr and that he bonded with you so well, but who doesn't??? You are the best! We love you and pray that the process will be getting easier. And of course STILL trying to make our way down.
> Andy, Heidi, Hayley & Cayden

3rd Chemo Treatment and Counting . . .
(2009-03-26 23:25) - Beth

We met with Dr. O. today and he was happy with the results, as well. After seeing the Doctor, Janny said, 'Never in my life would I expect to see you jump down from the table and say, 'Okay, time for chemo." I personally think she just appreciates the drugs that she's given in that IV. They call one of those bags 'red wine' and that seems to be how it hits her. Anyone that knows her knows she's not a drinker, so she's a cheap date. She gets pretty buzzed up after her treatment. Tonight she took a 5 1/2 hour nap after her chemo. I can't tell you how happy it makes me that she is not going through what she witnessed her Grandmother fighting during chemotherapy!!

So, she only has one more treatment of the 'hard stuff' then four treatments of Herceptin, which shouldn't even make her nauseous. The second round should be a breeze for her. She's been so brave and strong. I can't begin to tell you how proud I am of her!

We had a really nice girls' night last night. Janny came over and we laughed and my mom made the best dinner ever!! She made a new recipe which was chicken piccata and roasted red potatoes and green beans. We finished everything but the beans. Oh my goodness, my mom was so stressed about it because we had never tried this recipe, but it was such an incredible meal and time. We hadn't seen Janny since mom's last chemo appointment so it was nice to spend some quality time with her again!!

As you can see I've been taking some pictures relating to cancer. I will throw them in here and there and I hope they're not too dramatic for you, but this IS our life now!!

2009 April

You're not going to believe this!
(2009-04-01 18:27) - Beth

Guess what?! I hit the lotto last night and now I can fund *project: 'I am Beautiful'* myself. Isn't that the most incredible news you've ever heard???

APRIL FOOLS!

Well, sort of because I do plan to hit the lotto tonight and fund the project myself although I am meeting with a woman on Friday who is a 12-year breast cancer survivor and has been a fundraiser for years and she is really high on this entire idea. I'm sure I'll have people throwing money at me to be involved with this and if they feel that passionate about it, how can I take that away from them?! I know for a fact it makes you feel good to do good for other people. It almost feels selfish because it makes me feel so good that it's almost as if I am doing it for myself. Perhaps that's just an added perk of doing nice things for others is that it makes everyone feel good!

So, everyone get out there and do good deeds. It can be as simple as a smile to someone that really needs one! And something else that I learned somewhere along the way if someone is rude to you, don't get mad, but just wonder what happened to them to put them into that rude state of mind. I like to tell people 'I'm sorry they're having a bad day!' That usually changes their mood instantly and I haven't gotten punched... yet!

Mom is feeling pretty lousy lately, but she will blog again when she is feeling better.

Have a good deed day!

Feeling Helpless (2009-04-02 00:31) - Beth

Today didn't turn out anything like it was planned. I was supposed to do a virtual tour in Tampa, but that was canceled due to cloudy skies. People seem to want beautiful blue skies in their tours rather than white, overcast skies. Go figure. I had planned to take a friend with me to see how the whole process works as he is looking for other work because he hates what he is doing. Therefore, mom planned to make dinner for all of us upon our return.

She was making beef stew, which had to begin in the morning and cook all day. As she was prepping the meal, she began feeling very weak and shaky. Her legs and hands were shaky and she felt nauseous. Since the tour was canceled, I helped her with the prep and dishes. By the time we were done with the prep she told me she didn't even know if she could eat the dinner with us. A big disappointment!

My friend came over for dinner despite the fact that the tour was canceled because we had already prepared all this food. Mom stayed in her room the entire time. I felt guilty for having some fun when she was feeling so bad. I checked on her several times and she assured me there was nothing I could do for her. What an incredible feeling of helplessness! If I could take this all away from her and put it on myself, I would do it in a heartbeat. I absolutely HATE seeing her in pain and suffering. And I know her, and I'm guessing she is not even showing me half of what she is feeling because she doesn't want to upset me. It feels like my heart is literally breaking watching her go through all of this and trying to be a strong little soldier all by herself. I know that she knows I am here by her side always, but I also know that she is as stubborn as I am (she raised me that way) and doesn't want to burden me with the real pain she is feeling. Please God, if you're listening, let something really great come from this horrendous experience!!

> jmcastro88 (2009-04-10 23:41:00)
> I know how you feel, B., I wish I could take away her pain, physical and emotional, as well as take away yours. But the good news is that something good has already come of this. You guys are even closer than ever (if that's possible) - as are the three of us, and that's very important. Also, you've learned to appreciate the time we have and not to waste a minute of it. Life tends to come at us so quickly that we sometimes forget to think about what is really precious in life. Anyway, I think I might be babbling, so let me just end by saying that I love you both and am praying my head off for you. Let me know if there's anything you girls need and I'll see you on Wednesday for Girls' Night In!

Do you smell that? (2009-04-04 08:00) - CJ

I received the following email from my friends, Bob and Joan. I know some of you have seen it before but it is definitely worth another read.

In Dallas, the doctor walked into the small hospital room of Diana Blessing. She was still groggy from surgery. Her husband, David, held her hand as they braced themselves for the latest news.

That afternoon of March 10, 1991, complications had forced Diana, only 24-weeks pregnant, to undergo an emergency Cesarean to deliver the couple's new daughter, Dana Lu Blessing. At 12 inches long and weighing only one pound nine ounces, they already knew she was perilously premature.

Still, the doctor's soft words dropped like bombs. 'I don't think she's going to make it,' he said, as kindly as he could. 'There's only a 10-percent chance she will live through the night, and even then, if by some slim chance she does make it, her future could be a very cruel one.'

Numb with disbelief, David and Diana listened as the doctor described the devastating problems Dana would likely face if she survived.

She would never walk, she would never talk, she would probably be blind, and she would certainly be prone to other catastrophic conditions from cerebral palsy to complete mental retardation, and on and on.

'No! No!' was all Diana could say. She and David, with their 5-year-old son Dustin, had long dreamed of the day that they would have a daughter to become a family of four. Now, within a matter of hours, that dream was slipping away.

But as those first days passed, a new agony set in for David and Diana. Because Dana's underdeveloped nervous system was essentially 'raw', the lightest kiss or caress only intensified her discomfort, so they couldn't even cradle their tiny baby girl against their chests to offer the strength of their love. All they could do, as Dana struggled alone beneath the ultraviolet light in the tangle of tubes and wires, was to pray that God would stay close to their precious little girl.

There was never a moment when Dana suddenly grew stronger. But as the weeks went by, she did slowly gain an ounce of weight here and an ounce of strength there. At last, when Dana turned two months old, her parents were able to hold her in their arms for the very first time.

And two months later, though doctors continued to gently, but grimly, warn that her chances of surviving, much less living any kind of normal life, were next to zero, Dana went home from the hospital, just as her mother had predicted.

Five years later, Dana was a petite but feisty young girl with glittering gray eyes and an unquenchable zest for life. She showed no signs whatsoever of any mental or physical impairment. Simply, she was everything a little girl can be and more. But that happy ending is far from the end of her story.

One blistering afternoon in the summer of 1996, near her home in Irving, Texas, Dana was sitting in her mother's lap in the bleachers of a local ballpark where her brother Dustin's baseball team was practicing.

As always, Dana was chattering nonstop with her mother and several other adults sitting nearby when she suddenly fell silent. Hugging her arms across her chest, little Dana asked, 'Do you smell that?'

Smelling the air and detecting the approach of a thunderstorm, Diana replied, 'Yes, it smells like rain.'

Dana closed her eyes and again asked, 'Do you smell that?' Once again, her mother replied, 'Yes, I think we're about to get wet. It smells like rain.'

Still caught in the moment, Dana shook her head, patted her thin shoulders with her small hands and loudly announced, 'No, it smells like Him. It smells like God when you lay your head on His chest.'

Tears blurred Diana's eyes as Dana happily hopped down to play with the other children.

Before the rains came, her daughter's words confirmed what Diana and all the members of the extended Blessing family had known, at least in their hearts, all along.

During those long days and nights of her first two months of her life, when her nerves were too sensitive for them to touch her, God was holding Dana on His chest and it is His loving scent that she remembers so well.

Now, I don't know if this happens to anyone else (except my sister), but when I am getting sick, I smell weird smells. When I was pregnant, I was nauseous practically the whole nine months and I constantly smelled butterscotch. To this day, I can't stand the smell of butterscotch!

Anyhow, lately I have walked through a room and caught the sweet scent of flowers, mostly roses, or the comforting smell of my dad's aftershave. I choose to think it's God sending my guardian angels to check up on me!

Thank you all for your prayers and support!

Truth be told . . . I ache (2009-04-05 03:14) - Beth

I think I've been really strong throughout this entire journey thus far, but I think the time has come to share what is going on inside me right now.

I have no idea what is going to happen from one day to the next. I feel as though I am losing my strength, at least for the moment. I think I'm entitled to that. Now is that time.

I just need someone to hold me tight and tell me that everything is going to be alright . . . and MEAN IT!! I am desperately holding onto faith, but it doesn't seem to be pulling me through it right now.

And do you even know how many people go through it alone? It's heartbreaking! I can't bear to see that with anyone. You have to hold their hands, pick up their canes, and help them out of their chairs . . . whatever you have to do to make them feel they are not alone.

Truth be told . . . I ache! It hurts on the inside and outside. My chest hurts, my back throbs, my legs feel like they can no longer hold me up and then I begin to feel guilty because I am complaining when I can't even imagine what my mom is going through!!

Never mind, I am just allowing myself to 'feel' publicly, for a change. I try to be strong for everyone. I just wanted to take a moment to let myself be free to feel and I wanted to be honest about it.

Anyway, I have high hopes that everything is going to turn out perfect, but please continue to pray for us! We love you all!

Feeling Better (2009-04-05 23:55) - CJ

Finally, I am feeling a little better. Since I have last updated everyone, I have been to see Dr. S. for my post-op exam, as well as Dr. O. for my regular bi-weekly exam. They both agree, and are delighted, that the chemo is doing its job. The tumor has shrunk significantly. The pain has abated as my skin is no longer being stretched beyond its limits.

The 'red devil' really kicked my butt this time. I was able to eat very little and lost six pounds in one week.

I've been on tons of diets in my life and have never lost that much in that time before! So when I went for blood work my counts were down and they gave me additional IV fluids, which did make me feel somewhat better. At least I was able to eat a little more.

I just get so tired. I tried to make dinner the other night and was only able to do that with Beth's help. I just don't know what I would do without her! I feel so bad when we go to the doctors and see so many people going through this alone. And Beth is always there; ready to help them, as well.

If I'm trying to do something around the house, I have to work for twenty minutes or so, and then take a rest. As you might imagine, at that rate, it takes quite a long time to get things done.

The good thing is that I only have one more dose of that damn red devil, and then will switch meds for the second course of chemo.

And Dr. O. tells me that the second course doesn't make people nauseous, thank goodness!

Beth, Janice and I have reserved the Wednesday night before my chemo appointments as 'girls' night in' since that's the day I usually feel the best. I really look forward to these nights and love that time that I get to spend with them. We usually don't even talk about cancer, just laugh and carry on like we don't have a care in the world, and believe me, we all need that!

So, for all of you to whom I owe phone calls, please be patient. I just haven't had the strength lately to even talk on the phone. Please continue to follow the blog (and comment!) and please continue to keep us in your prayers.

We love you all and thank you all so much for your prayers and support!

Thanks Janny! (2009-04-09 22:40) - Beth

I just wanted to thank you again for the other night. We really had fun and needed it. I told my mom before you came over that I might just cry all night. I've been really weepy lately for some reason. She said, 'Then do what you need to do' and I never once felt the desire to cry. It feels so good to laugh that hard and you know, none of us have the good sense that God gave us! I guess what I'm saying is 'Thanks for being there for us!!'

We Love You!

> jmcastro88 (2009-04-10 07:20:00)
> Well, you are certainly welcome, but no thanks are necessary. I look forward to our girls' nights more than you can know. And anytime you feel weepy and need a shoulder, mine is available.
> Also, I want to thank you for the conversation the other day (a day that wasn't today) and allowing me to vent to you. I love you "skanklettes"!!!

Anonymous (2009-04-16 16:11:00)
Umm, someone needs to find their own words-don't be stealing mine girl. LOL, I love all of you little skanklettes.

Art by Beth (2009-04-16 23:25:00)
For someone that wants to claim words they made up . . . why did you sign it 'anonymous'??
We love you too and I hope you 'skanklettes' (property of Lisa D.) have fun this weekend!

The Last 'Red Devil' (2009-04-12 06:11) - CJ

I almost titled this 'Red Devil be damned' until I realized it did exactly what it's supposed to do...shrink the tumor. When we started this journey, obsessive-compulsive that I am, I broke it down into sections...finding a team of doctors, testing, port implant surgery, red devil chemo, Herceptin chemo, radiation, mastectomy, and more Herceptin chemo. The good news is that I am now halfway through!

I saw Dr. O. on Thursday before my last dose of the red devil and he is very pleased with the results of the chemo. He assured me that the next round will not make me sick and if it does, says I can throw things at him. He did, however, specify that the 'things' have to be styrofoam balls!

I fell asleep while I was having my chemo and when I woke up, Beth and Janice said they were making fun of me like I wasn't even there! Oh well, if they're making fun of me, they're leaving someone else alone!

I had my Neulasta shot on Friday and am starting to feel the effects of the chemo today, the shakiness and weakness, loss of appetite and just plain tired, from my white count being low. On Tuesday I go for a routine echocardiogram to make sure my heart function isn't being affected by the chemo.

Beth and Janice...I want you both to know how very important you have been so far throughout this journey. Believe me when I say I couldn't, and wouldn't, have done this without the two of you. You respected my initial decision to not have treatment, but somehow gently convinced me that was what I needed to do. You have cried with me, and more importantly, laughed with me! You both seem to know what I need and exactly when I need it and there is no 'thank you' big enough for that! You really are my angels and I love you more than you know!! THANK YOU, THANK YOU, THANK YOU!

Another side effect (2009-04-15 07:12) - CJ

I had been feeling weak and shaky since Sunday. When we went for my ECHO on Tuesday (results still unknown), we stopped at Dr. O's office for an unscheduled visit to see why. I thought they would just give me additional fluids as they have before and all would be well. However, they didn't quite understand the reason for the weakness. I was hydrated, I was eating, my blood sugar was good, no nausea or stomach pain. But when they ran my blood work, it seems that my hemoglobin was dangerously low. It should be in the 12.0 to 17.0 range and it was 9.5, making me anemic. They said that if it dropped to 9.0, I would have needed a transfusion, so I'm glad that we didn't wait till my regular appointment on Thursday. They gave me a shot along with the fluids to build my hemoglobin back up and said the only side effects would be good ones...that I would start to feel better. I guess I was looking for more instantaneous gratification and was disappointed that I still wasn't feeling much better by the time we got home, about six hours later.

Beth and I had both had bad nights, sleeping poorly and nightmares, we were having serious thunderstorms all day and we decided to call it a day. Close the blinds and take naps. That only worked for one of us. I was seriously moody because I couldn't sleep, even with a little help from my 'friends'. I ended up not falling asleep until after 1:00 a.m., having been up since 4:00 a.m. the previous day! I do seem to be feeling somewhat better today, so hopefully, the shot is doing its thing.

The bad news is that the new chemo may have this same result, so I'm sure that is another thing they will monitor closely now. However, I do consider myself lucky that I have bypassed (knock wood!) some of the more serious side effects of the chemo. I will start my new chemo regime on April 23 and look forward to the downhill slope of this journey!

Thank you all for your prayers and support!

> Anonymous (2009-04-19 16:30:00)
> Carol and Beth
> I have been following your blog pretty regularly and have tried to comment a few times but, screwed up the end and lost my text (you think I would at least know how to post a blog comment - - NOT). Anyway, I want to commend both of you on your strength and courage and to let you know that our prayers and thoughts are with you throughout this journey (which will be successful). Your ups and downs are to be expected but because of the love you two share, you continue on. Good news and bad news - - you continue on - - one living and being strong for the other (not wanting to let the other one down). Continue on, continue on. Your journey will take you and your love to places neither has been. Please keep the blog going. It is a good thing for all of us. Be strong and continue on knowing that many share your love.
> Mike P.

More 'thank you's' (2009-04-18 09:28) - CJ

Beth and I count our blessings every day and one of the biggest is the great support network of family and friends we have!

Rich...thanks for the check. We appreciate it more than you know. Thanks also for the inspiring emails and for your prayers!

Dennis and Michelle...thanks for the cards and the check. I always love hearing from you guys and hope to connect with you by phone sometime soon! Your card to Beth was especially heart-warming when she is going through such a hard time!

'Mom'...thanks for the cards and your gift of cash. I know you are going through your own health issues and I appreciate you and miss you so much!

Brett...thanks for the card and your gift of cash. It means a lot to us and will be put to good use.

Mario...thanks for coming over on Easter and making us dinner...Beef Wellington and sautéed asparagus...YUMMY!

My own personal HUGE thank you to Beth and Jan, as always, for being by my side every step of the way throughout this journey! What would I do without you guys?!!! I love you both more than you know!

I hope I haven't missed anyone on this latest round of gratitude. Please continue to keep up with the blog and to keep us in your prayers, as we do you.

Wow . . . almost two weeks (2009-04-22 00:31) - Beth

Wow, I just realized it's been almost two weeks since I've blogged. Sorry! I've been busy and stressed lately and I didn't really want that to reflect in my blog. I know this is supposed to be all about honesty, but honestly, I didn't want to be negative!

So, I've been working feverishly on the *project: 'I am Beautiful'* website. I added some images of 'My Inspiration' for the entire idea. I purchased www.projectIamBeautiful.org and .com and redirected those to the site I currently have designed. Once I have obtained funding, I will have the site redesigned to be much more interactive and user-friendly.

I also contacted 16 celebrity contacts (i.e., agents, managers, publicists) that support breast cancer charities for their endorsements, funding, publicity, and items they are able to donate for future fundraisers in honor of this project. I have about 135 celebrities left to contact, but I need to obtain additional information for the initial contact. Wow, this stuff takes a lot of time and effort, but I really feel that this endeavor is going to pay off tremendously. I believe this is my personal mission in life. As hard as some things are to deal with, I feel this is why my mother was diagnosed with breast cancer. Because this is something that is not out there and needs to be!!

On another note, I was very concerned when I found out about mom's hemoglobin being so down that she could have potentially needed a blood transfusion. I don't really know much about that, but it just sounds really frightening.

I didn't have quite as hard a time with her second Echo as I did the first one. I know they are just doing it for safety sake this time. That first time though, as I mentioned then, I was literally watching her heart beating and I couldn't even imagine it stopping the thump, thump, thumping. The thought of that brought me to a screeching halt. She's my whole world and I love her more than life itself!!

We are continuing on this journey and, I believe, we will get through this and have found our mission in life, in the meantime.

Thank you all for your prayers, your inspiration, and your support! Please keep the prayers coming. It is not an easy journey, but I feel we will prevail and offer much support for others that have gone through the same or who will travel a similar path!!

New chemo (2009-04-24 09:33) - CJ

I went to see Dr. O. yesterday and my ECHO was fine. He is very pleased that the tumor has shrunk to one-third of its former size and is definitely not attached to the chest wall. He assured me once again that the new chemo would not cause nausea and I assured him that if it does, the next time I see him I would bring Styrofoam balls to throw at him, per his former suggestion!

We head back to the chemo room where I'm settled in and my blood work is run. My hemoglobin is even lower now, 8.9, but Dr. O. opts for no blood transfusion at this point since I am not feeling weak or shaky, and will monitor it closely. He says the shot I got last Tuesday sometimes takes a couple weeks to build me back up.

The new chemo consists of Herceptin, which is believed to: block the ability of tumor cells to grow and divide, to signal the body's immune system that abnormal cells (tumor cells) are present so that certain immune system cells can attack the tumor cells and work in conjunction with chemotherapy to slow the growth of tumors. It also includes Taxol, which slows or stops the growth of cancer cells in the body. I get my regular pre-meds with it, which include Benadryl and Ativan, the ones that make me 'loopy', the ones I like!

I dozed off pretty much immediately, since I had been awake since 3:45 a.m., and apparently, the girls sat and made fun of me, sweet little things that they are! When I woke, I told them they didn't have to stay as this treatment takes three to five hours, but they wouldn't hear of it. We finally were good to go at 4:40 p.m. (from 9:50 a.m.)! It really IS a full-time job, unfortunately, one that you don't get paid for.

After some dinner, I slept pretty much the rest of the evening, waking at about 11:30 p.m. to tell Beth and Roxy good-night!

This morning I go for my Neulasta shot and, so far, am feeling pretty decent.

Dreams really do come true! (2009-04-30 18:59) - Beth

How many times a day when you look at someone, you automatically place them into a category? It doesn't have to be a negative thing. For example, you turn around at the bookstore and suddenly, you've caught a glimpse of his eyes (and other things) as he does you and there is this strange electric current running between the two of you for just a minute. You then immediately place him in the 'eye candy' category . . . not a bad place to be! This is actually a true story!!

Anyway, on a lighter note, I was contacted by a friend that I went to school with on Facebook but hadn't heard from in 21 years. He lives in the area and we got together for dinner and drinks the other night. I had such a great time talking with someone that I've known for a long time, but haven't 'known for a long time' (and somehow this really makes sense). We talked about old times and the times that we didn't 'know' each other. We had a lot of laughs and that is what the doctor ordered!

In addition, I found out that cousin Mike is coming for a visit the weekend of May 15th. For those of you that don't know (although he will deny it), Mike was my mentor. He gave me the strength to do the traveling circus, er, I mean, legal thing. I could use some of that 'strength' about now!

Mom's second round of treatment is kicking her butt more than the first round. We thought it was going to be easier on her this time around. I guess we have to go to her next oncology appointment with Styrofoam balls!!

This blog has gone in all different directions, but my real point was . . . don't judge a book by its cover. And dreams really do come true so hold on to them, believe they will happen and they will!

2009 May

Apologies (2009-05-09 07:45) - CJ

I apologize to all for not having posted in so long, but the new chemo kicked my butt! I had LOTS of bone and joint pain and was really miserable. I saw Dr. O. on Thursday and he thinks the pain may have been caused by the Neulasta. Since the new chemo doesn't affect my white count, we will try going without the Neulasta this week. Next week when I go for my blood work, if my white count is down, they will give me a shot. But, the good news is that the tumor has shrunk significantly! He hopes the new chemo will continue to shrink it even more. I only have two more treatments, so he is predicting my surgery for some time in July. I see Dr. S. on May 14, so I will know more then. That's pretty scary now that it is looming closer. I am feeling more depressed and I think that's why. I am having a hard time sleeping and lots of nightmares so; consequently, I am fatigued all day.

Of course, we had 'girls' night in' Wednesday night and a good time was had by all, as usual. And the girls continue to make fun of me when I go to sleep during chemo so there are still lots of laughs!

So far, no side effects from the latest chemo, except that my hemoglobin is still low, so they gave me a shot of Aranesp to build me back up. The weird thing about that is that it makes my lips numb for a couple days. Dr. O. said I'm the first one who has told him that...leave it to me!

So, yes, I'm still hanging in there and on the downward slope, not looking forward to the surgery, but definitely looking forward to being cancer-free!

Thanks to all for your prayers and support!

I promise myself (2009-05-11 22:40) - Beth

This is a piece I came upon a while ago and printed it out. I intended to read it the minute I awoke every morning, but that never happened. I think it is beautiful and I am going to place it on my nightstand and 'promise myself' to read it every morning! I suggest you all do the same and let's see if it makes a difference in our day. Deal?

I promise myself . . .

To be so strong that nothing can disturb my peace of mind.

To talk health, happiness, and prosperity to every person I meet.

To make all my friends feel
that there is something worthwhile in them.

To look at the sunny side of everything
and make my optimism come true.

To think only of the best, to work only for the best
and to expect only the best.

To be just as enthusiastic about the success of others
as I am about my own.

To forget the mistakes of the past and press on
to the greater achievements of the future.

To wear a cheerful expression at all times
and give a smile to every living creature I meet.

To give so much time to improving myself
that I have no time to criticize others.
To be too large for worry, too noble for anger, too strong for fear
and too happy to permit the presence of trouble.
To think well of myself and to proclaim this fact to the world,
not in loud words, but in great deeds.
To live in faith that the whole world is on my side,
so long as I am true to the best that is in me.
Christian D. Larson Modified by The Secret

Hyatt 365 free nights (2009-05-12 14:04) - Beth

Hyatt is holding an essay contest on how one would create an unforgettable experience with 365 free nights at Hyatt along with 1 million frequent flyer miles.

Below is my submission:

I would create an unforgettable experience with my 365 free nights at Hyatt by giving away the experience to other women. Please, let me explain...

After my mother's recent diagnosis of breast cancer and taking this journey with her in battling this deadly disease, it's become my mission to help these women feel beautiful again! My desire is to create a Fine Art, intimate photography book of their lovely bodies.

Women dealing with breast cancer have many things to worry about, from juggling everyday family life to time off work, while healing from this deadly disease. In addition, they grieve the loss of all things 'womanly' about their personal appearance, leaving a feeling of hopelessness.

Another serious problem, particularly during this economic crisis, cancer doesn't wait until you are financially secure to strike.

People are struggling to keep their jobs and homes, but women continue to be told every day that they have breast cancer. Stress isn't kind to women struggling to fight for their lives. Increasing funding for financial assistance to women healing from breast cancer will allow these women to concentrate solely on healing, physically and emotionally.

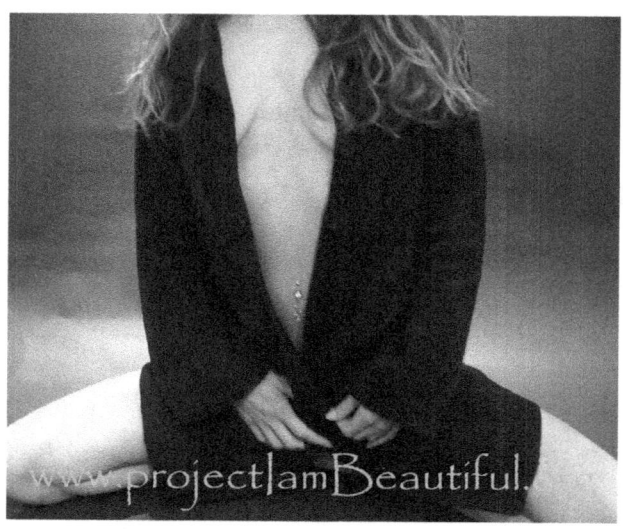

My vision is to obtain funding for the project so proceeds from the book will go towards non-medical financial assistance (mortgage, utilities, etc.)

For this reason, I would give my experience to other women in order for them to be included in this very special opportunity where they can announce to the world… 'I am Beautiful'

They will notify the Top 20 semi-finalists on May 15th, consumers will vote for Top 5 finalists during May 26th - June 2nd and the Grand Prize Winner will be announced June 12th. So, send out all your good karma and let's get this project started!!

"drive-through" mastectomies (2009-05-13 02:01) - Beth

The Bipartisan Breast Cancer Patient Protection Act Needs Your Support!

This week Representatives Rosa DeLauro (D-Connecticut) and Joe Barton (R-Texas) and Senators Mary Landrieu (D-Louisiana) and Olympia Snowe (R-Maine) will re-introduce the bipartisan Breast Cancer Patient Protection Act in Congress. Thanks to its viewers, Lifetime has so far collected more than 23 million online petition signatures urging Congress to pass this critical legislation, which would end the practice of so-called "drive-through" mastectomies when women are forced out of the hospital only hours after invasive breast cancer surgery.

I spoke too soon! (2009-05-13 11:51) - CJ

Me and my big, fat mouth! Saturday afternoon the bone and joint pain hit with a vengeance and has not yet abated, in spite of various meds. Clearly, it is the Taxol and not the Neulasta that is causing the pain because I didn't have the Neulasta last week. I have to say I really think it is worse than the 'red devil'...and this is supposed to be the easy one! It is so difficult to do anything, even walking from room to room, that I pretty much just lie on the couch, sleeping whenever possible. Even then, the pain can wake me from sleep. What was I thinking when I said I was now on the downward slope?!! Oh well, only two more treatments...surely I can get through that!

Pre-Op Appointment (2009-05-15 22:27) - Beth

Today we had a follow-up appointment, but turns out it was really more like a 'pre-op' appointment. Mom's not looking forward to mastectomy day (and you can't really blame her)! She's been a champ throughout this entire journey, so far, and I just can't tell you how proud of her I am!! She really is my Hero.

An Epiphany (2009-05-20 16:18) - Beth

Wow, I was playing with my little dog and she wanted to play tug. She was getting it in her mouth just right when I tugged and won the toy. She looked at me with those big brown eyes as if to say, "Hey, I wasn't ready yet." And I spoke to her (as I often do) and told her, "Roxy, life doesn't wait to start until you get a grip."

At that moment it hit me like a ton of bricks. I have to get a grip on life because it's not going to wait for me either. So, life dealt me a really crappy hand right now, but I have to get a grip and deal with it. Obviously, my life would be a lot better if cancer wasn't in it; if my best friend was healthy and happy! And then there's the recession. Would it have been easier had cancer and the recession not shown up at my door hand in hand, of course! Unfortunately, that is not the case here.

I need to pull myself up by my bootstraps (yes, I wear boots in Florida) and deal with the obstacles that life is placing in my path. I am working on some additional ideas as we speak and I'm sure that the Universe, the big guy/girl, karma or whatever is supposed to be watching my back and being my spiritual adviser is going to help me through it.

Anyway, we should really listen to the advice we give to others because chances are . . . it is the very advice we should be heeding ourselves!

Taxol, be damned! (2009-05-22 09:19) - CJ

I went to see Dr. S. last Friday. As usual, he gave me a big hug...Dr. Rude sure could take lessons from him in 'Bedside Manner'!! Needless to say, he is very pleased with the size of the tumor. He will do my surgery the end of June or the beginning of July. We discussed my having both breasts removed because I really don't want to go through this again. He made the case for both sides and said he will do whatever I want. I am leaning toward bilateral but can change my mind up until surgery.

The bone and joint pain and the neuropathy in my feet are nearly unbearable. I went for my appointment with Dr. O. yesterday. He said he has been watching my liver enzymes and they have risen 400-500 % since I have been on the Taxol...NOT good. It is called chemical hepatitis, which will go away once I am off the Taxol. Because of that and the pain and neuropathy, he will start giving me partial doses but I will get them every week instead of bi-weekly. I had the first one yesterday and it was about two hours shorter than normal because of the lower dose. All the nurses there are so kind. No matter how many people are there, no matter how many machines are 'beeping' to be changed, they are never too busy to answer questions or to give support and a compassionate word. They really do get to be like family.

So yeah, I was very lucky not to have all the bad side effects of the 'red devil', but the Taxol sure is getting revenge. Thankfully, only four more weeks of it, and hopefully, the lower dose will make a difference. Please keep those prayers coming...we sure can use them! I love you all and thanks so very much for all your support!

The Vine . . . (2009-05-28 21:28) - Beth

It's been raining here, pretty much, non-stop for a couple of weeks now. I was out front pulling mushrooms from my front yard twice this week.' I wish I could find a way to profit from those mushrooms growing!

There are vines in my backyard that I endlessly attempt to eliminate and they continue to grow regardless of my efforts to thwart them. Tonight though, I took a moment to appreciate the beauty in them. The sky was a beautiful blue and the vine . . . a vibrant red. I had to get up out of my seat to really see the vision, but it was definitely worth the trip!

I felt the need to run inside to grab my camera and capture the moment forever. If you think about it, the moment you are living will never happen again in anyone's lifetime. I think that's what makes every moment so very precious!

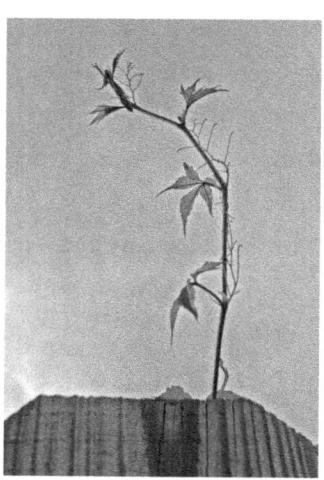

Tomorrow, I will be back on my mission of eliminating the vine that will eventually pull my fence down upon growing large enough, but I will embrace the beauty of the vine . . . in the moment!

. . . three things (2009-05-28 22:38) - CJ

I went for my chemo again today, with my angels, Beth and Janice, in tow. Thanks, girls!! And after chemo, Janice took us to lunch. Thanks, James!! My hemoglobin's continue to rise and are just .5 from being normal. The chemo only lasted three hours, including about a 20-minute wait for the hook-up and blood work. The lower dose is definitely making a difference in the pain...it's still there but bearable. I'm sure Dr. O. will update me on the liver enzymes next Thursday when I see him.

The chemo routine, strange as it may sound, has almost become a comfort zone for me. We have gotten to know several of the patients, and the nurses are like family. We all share cancer stories and jokes. Thank goodness for the jokes because the cancer stories are pretty grim sometimes. We talked with a woman today who has three children, 7, 8 and 12. She got colon cancer in 2006 and they removed about a foot of her colon. It has now returned and is in her liver and lungs, and there is no surgery they can do to 'fix' her. Several weeks ago, her port failed and she had to have it removed and replaced. Every couple weeks she has to go home from chemo with a pump attached to her port overnight and return the next day to have it removed. Last week her red cells were down to 6 and she had to have four units of blood over two days. Her company laid her off since she has to have appointments each Thursday and Friday, but she can't collect unemployment because she's not 'looking for work'. She said she is living for her kids and continues to get them to their dance classes, sports, and other activities. And then, as if on cue, 'Missy, the mean nurse' comes through saying that ZZ Top is in the Nautical (blood work) Room! Of course, Beth and Janice had to go over to see. They said 'could have been', but they weren't really sure!

...and the second thing...maybe the chemo is my comfort zone because of the upcoming surgery, currently scheduled for July 1? I know you're reading this, Dr. S., whaddya' think? I am so unbelievably petrified and, in all honesty, don't know if I can go through with it. Beth and I were talking with a woman the other day who had her surgery in February. She got lymphedema and was giving me tips to avoid it. She really was being helpful, not morbid, but I had to tell her to stop, that I was getting sick to my stomach and I had to go and sit down. Of course, she felt horrible when Beth told her how terrified I am and she came over to give me a hug and some words of comfort. I just think of it and begin to cry. I know, I know, I was afraid of the port implant and biopsies and got through that, I was afraid of the chemo and got through that, but this is huge. I have said, 'What difference does it make. I'm 61 and don't really need them'. Everything I have heard and read says it is a grieving process, that you will mourn the loss of a body part. But when I think of waking up to look down and see nothing, I just don't think I can do it. I feel guilty when I watch or hear of stories of young women just starting their lives, or in the prime of them, getting cancer, or of women who are pregnant getting it, but that doesn't make my fear any less real. People tell me that I am brave and I feel like a fraud.

I'm sure our situation isn't helping. Those of you who have known Beth and me forever know that we have been in some pretty grim spots, but believe me when I say this is the grimmest. I feel that God has deserted us and for the first time in my life, feel completely hopeless. I'm certain most of you will tell me to go back and read what I have written, that things could be way worse and I know that's true, but that really doesn't help when we are struggling every day to try to figure out how we are going to earn an income. Sure, lots of people are struggling in today's economy and I do have compassion for them but, in all honesty, and I'm sorry if this sounds selfish, we don't have to pay their bills. I fear the toll it is taking on Beth because the load is all on her. In the 'old days', even at my age, with good health I could go out and 'sling hash'. Not anymore...never mind the good health part, look how many restaurants have closed down.

I know that my blogs have been pretty cut and dried lately. That's because I have been keeping everything bottled up and not being honest and that's not the purpose of this blog. This one's not pretty, but it's real.

A Small Price to Pay . . . (2009-05-31 00:11) - Beth

We have talked about this since we both learned of her cancer, but for some reason, hadn't yet done it. Today we got our pink ribbon tattoo!! Janny got hers on her outer right ankle and I got mine on the inner left ankle. Yes, it hurt like hell, but it was worth it to honor my mom! Janny and I were like little kids keeping a secret from her . . . giggling and all.

Today was the day that mom told me she would go through with the surgery 'for me', so in my mind, today was the day to honor 'her'. Funny thing was, Janny texted me wanting to know if today was 'tattoo day' before she even talked to my mom. And after mom told her that she decided to go through with the surgery, she knew in her heart of hearts too.

When the discussion first came up, I thought I would get the tattoo on the same breast of my mother's cancer. After hearing her discuss her confusion over taking something foreign out of your breast and then introducing something new (i.e., a tattooed nipple) . . . that might not be the best thing to do. I'd since re-thought the location of my tat. Once I decided on my ankle, I couldn't decide on the inner or outer side. I thought I could better protect on the inside, so that's what I chose to do. I want to protect her and I shall!

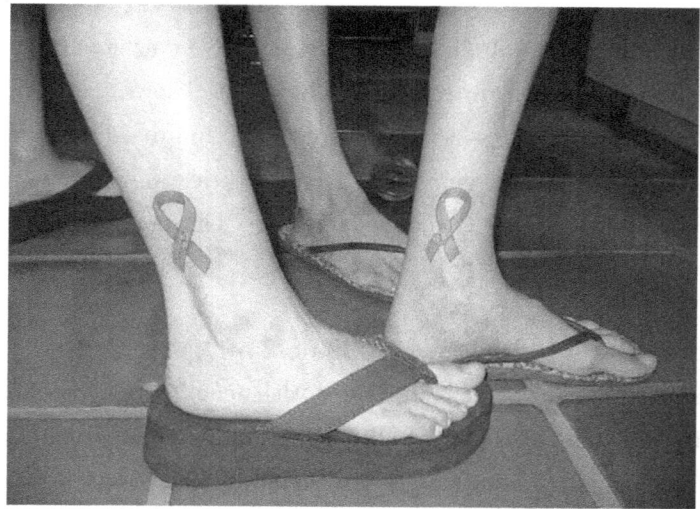

When we showed her our surprise, she felt much honored and spoke of such. She is the reason I live! I feel this is a small price to pay for what she is doing for me!! I love you so much, Ma!

2009 June

My posse ROCKS!!! (2009-06-04 21:06) - CJ

On Saturday, Beth and Jan made plans to go out for a drink early evening. They did, and a couple hours later called to say that they were going to pick up Lauren, my niece, and come over, that they had a surprise for me. I thought it was probably food, specifically, nachos and cheese from the VIP. So they come and they are both stooped down, I thought playing with Roxy, and acting weird, nothing unusual so it took me awhile to figure it was a little TOO weird and a little TOO long. They giggled when I asked them what they were up to and stood up and showed me their ankles! My first response was, 'Those are fake!' I know how much Beth's first one hurt and was convinced she wouldn't go through it again, and for some strange reason, as long as I have known my 'seester', I never knew she wanted a tattoo! I mean, Dr. Castro can't even watch them put the needle in my port!

I was very honored that they had done it, and if I wasn't such a nut job lately from the fear of the surgery, I would have been in a heap on the floor, sobbing! Even five days later and they are still in pain, poor things. Girls, this is one of the nicest things anyone has ever done for me and it means SO much to me. Thank you both very much and I love you both more than you know.

And, as Beth said in her blog, THAT was the day that I actually decided I would go ahead with the surgery. Beth and I had been talking earlier in the day and she made a comment about 'you're going to leave me...' and I realized how totally selfish I was being. She was doing everything she could possibly do, and more, and I was ready to bail at this point, after already going through the testing and the chemo, after getting past the half-way point. At that instant, I told her I would have the surgery, that I don't want to leave her and can't bear to think of it. I love YOU so much, B. Later, when I talked with Janice on the phone, I told her about my decision and she said she was very glad, that she had been losing sleep over it. These two really have been my angels throughout this process, how could I possibly let them fight this hard for me and then give up? It was a no-brainer at that point, so girls, know that this is in honor of YOU!

I took homemade goodies to the chemo nurses today...those girls love to eat! Beth and Jan showed the first nurse their tattoos and I told her the story and pretty soon, the other nurses were coming in to see them. They all thought it was very cool!

I saw Dr. O today (totally forgot to show HIM the tats!) and he said my liver enzymes had dropped to a safe zone and my blood work showed that my hemoglobin's, though still not in range, were very good. I told him that the bone and joint pain was certainly tolerable at this point, so the half-dose every week is working. I have one more chemo treatment with the Taxol, and then I will continue to get the Herceptin IV every three weeks, starting 6/25, for a year. They claim there are no side effects with this one. I will have six weeks, five days a week, of radiation. But who knew that Dr. O. doesn't do this, so I have an appointment with a Radiation Oncologist, hereafter referred to as Dr. RO, on 7/22. They say the only side effect of the radiation, though it only takes two minutes, is fatigue. Dr. O. says less than chemo, the chemo nurses say more than chemo. On June 23, I have a pre-op appointment and the surgery has been rescheduled to July 8. On July 2, I will have my third follow-up ECHO.

Looks like the next two months are going to be pretty hectic, so please let me apologize in advance if the blog isn't as up-to-date as we would like it to be and I promise to do my best, as I'm sure, does Beth.

I am feeling better, physically and mentally, since I decided on the surgery. I felt paralyzed by indecision and couldn't manage to come up with too many things to be grateful for. That is coming a little easier these last few days, although I still have my moments...days.

Lauren is out of school now so she went with us today. Jan took us all to lunch after...thanks a bunch, James! We had a little room all to ourselves and we all got pink wristbands...HOPE, STRENGTH, BELIEVE, and SURVIVOR. I am starting to BELIEVE that there is HOPE now, and that, together with my angels and the continued prayers of my family and friends, I will have the STRENGTH to become a SURVIVOR.

Many thanks to all of you.

(We miss you and love you, Mom!)

Ponce816 (2009-06-09 10:13:09)
I am so glad to hear of your decision to have the surgery. I can't imagine what you went through while making this choice, but I know in my heart was the right one. You are a very strong person and I am very proud to be your brother. I want you to know that if there is anything I can do for you don't hesitate to let me know. You were my inspiration during my own ordeal and for that, I will be forever thankful. I love you and my prayers are with you always.
John

Don't mess with a momma's cub! (2009-06-11 21:45) - Beth

My mom did it!! Today was her last day of 'chemo'. She is a champ in my eyes. She didn't think she could get through it, but she did. I'm so proud of her!

The term is a little misleading because when I heard it, I thought it meant she was done seeing the chemo nurses. However, she still needs to go every three weeks to get Herceptin in IV form for a year before she will just take the Herceptin pill.

It seems that our roles have reversed since she has been diagnosed with breast cancer. It's as if she is my cub and I must care for her. As a matter of fact, Dr. Shrink told her the other day to tell me to stop treating her like a china doll. She is my little cub now and I don't want anyone messing with her!

On another, slightly humorous note: Times sure are changing. On the way home from chemo, we stopped to get gas. I was approached by a man asking if I had some change that he could put in his gas tank. I explained, 'I, too, was looking for work. Sorry.' He replied, 'You're too cute to even get mad at!' Did I just get hit on? Is that the 2009 version of a 'pick-up line'?

Would he actually 'get mad' if the person he had approached wasn't cute and didn't put gas in his vehicle? There was a man pumping gas behind me that this fellow didn't approach. Wasn't he 'cute' enough?

I've been around for a while so I can educationally say that pick-up lines have always started with a question: 'Can I buy you a drink?' 'Do you come here often?' 'You here alone?' But NEVER in my life have I heard the opening question be: 'Do you have some change to put in my gas tank?' In hindsight, I should have responded . . . 'Don't you think gas would run better?'

Anyway Ma, I think you should be proud of yourself because I know I am! All my heart!!

Bits 'n Pieces (2009-06-18 19:11) - CJ

Went for my blood work today and things are getting back to normal. The nurse told us that I will probably still have blood work every six weeks or so, now that I have finished my chemo...woo hoo!...and that some peoples' blood never gets quite back to normal.

I had to give Laura a hug before we left. She seemed to be a little frustrated from getting a lot of flak from a couple different patients and I wanted to support HER for a change. She is the nurse that has the little girl who had a rare type of cancer as an infant. She thanked me and said that I had made her day, which, in turn, made MY day.

I am feeling quite a bit better now and have been reassured that the Herceptin is a breeze. I am still scared about the surgery, as well as the recovery, which supposedly is NOT a breeze, but I guess if God gets me to it, He will get me through it. At least that's what I'm hoping!

We had girls' night in yesterday, which included Lauren this time, and actually started during the day so the girls could swim. It was lots of fun, as usual, and Roxy has made Lauren her new friend.

I go for my pre-op appointment on 6/23 and for my first Herceptin IV on 6/25 and will keep y'all posted. Thanks to Dennis and Michelle for the card and check and also thanks to Rich for the check! Thanks to all for your continued prayers and support. They have certainly gotten us through some of our darkest days.

On a lighter note, we have a new addition to our family...beautiful little Chloe Isabella Pauvlinch, born 6/17 to Andy and Heidi and baby sister to Hayley and Cayden. She was born a month early but is already out of the incubator and is spending time in her Mama's room. Welcome, little 'bella...we can't wait to see you!

Appointment updates (2009-06-26 11:32) - CJ

I want to start by thanking my sister-in-law, Kathy, for doing the Race for the Cure at Bradys Run Park back home in PA in my honor. As well as losing her husband, my brother, Ed, just a year ago, Kathy has had her own illnesses and health problems and is raising two sons on her own and yet, took the time to do this for me and for millions of other women with this disease. Thank you, Kath. I love you and appreciate it so much!!

Beth, Janice and I went for my pre-op appointment on Tuesday. We were sitting in the waiting room when Dr. S. popped his head in and waved. He was out in the hallway talking to some people and when he finished, he came in to give me a hug, as usual, and to chat a bit. We had a few questions for him and, unlike most doctors; he took his time giving us the answers we needed. I will have drainage tubes for two or three weeks, at which time they will be removed. One of the questions Beth had for him was how they are removed. With a perfectly serious look on his face, he said, 'we usually tie them to a doorknob and slam the door.' So I'm thinking if he's ever looking for a second job, comedian may be the ticket!

My surgery is still scheduled for July 8 at 7:15 a.m. Since I have to be there at 5:15, and since I will be in the hospital for two days, we have decided to stay at a hotel nearby the night before, thanks to the hotel points Beth accumulated when she was traveling so much. Beth and Jan will then stay until I am discharged. In addition, we will be able to take Roxy with us. She hates the kennel and doesn't eat when she is there, which is just another stressor for Beth.

I had my vitals taken and my medical history reviewed by Maria, who also happens to be a breast cancer survivor. She was very nice, answered lots of questions for us and, in general, put my mind at ease a little. I just had an EKG in January, so I didn't need another and since I have blood work when I go for my Herceptin, they will have that faxed to Dr. S., so it was quite an easy appointment.

Since we were done so early, we had another impromptu girls' day in and laughed even more than usual. I swear the three of us are too weird for color TV! Even Roxy was more comical than usual!

On Thursday, Beth and I went for my Herceptin. Janice didn't go because she, Joe and Lauren were taking a much-needed three-day trip. Hope you guys have a GREAT time!! Glad to say, no side effects at this point except that I was really tired when I got home and took a four-hour 'nap'.

The woman I wrote about a couple weeks ago who has three little ones and is fighting liver, lung and brain cancer, came in with a huge smile on her face and came over to tell us what great news she had that morning. She had had a PET scan and an MRI with fantastic results. The spot on her brain had shrunk significantly, and the spots on her liver and lung were gone completely! It's always good to hear that kind of story in the chemo room! We hugged her and told her how happy we were for her. They want her to do another three months of chemo, and she said she will GLADLY go through it.

There was another woman there who was having her first chemo treatment and was scared to death. I'm not sure what her story is, but chemo is chemo, and when they explain all the 'ins and outs' of it to you, it's frightening. Hopefully, hearing the good results of the other woman may help her through it. When we left, I told her to hang in there, that it really does get easier.

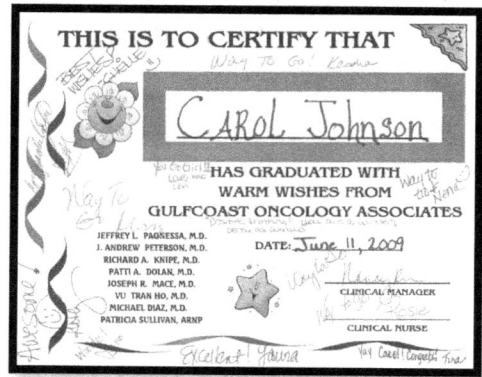

In addition, I got a certificate of 'graduation from chemo', signed by the nurses. As I was leaving, the nurses were congratulating and hugging me as we talked about what a mess I was when I first started. Some of the patients congratulated me and said, 'we are anxious to be where you are'. It's hard for me to believe that I am this far into it already. It seems like such a short time ago that I first told my family and was so adamant about not having treatment. Thank goodness for their support! In hindsight, it wasn't nearly as bad as I thought it would be and that's how I'm trying to think of the surgery, recovery, and radiation.

We love you all and thank you for your prayers and support!

2009 July

Benefit for Mom (2009-07-06 23:37) - Beth

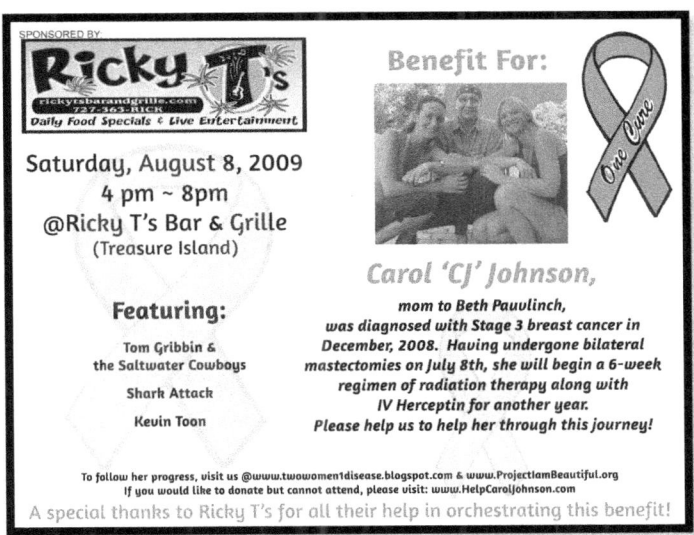

Oh my goodness, I'm so sorry it's been so long since I've blogged. There's been a lot going on lately. Janny & I started talking 'benefit' since we've found out about mom's breast cancer. She got the ball rolling several weeks ago. We met with the owner of Ricky T's Bar & Grille (my local watering hole)

twice now. They are going to sponsor the benefit and they are being very generous. We have the music line-up: Tom Gribbin & the Saltwater Cowboys, Shark Attack & Kevin Toon. We are even working towards a guest appearance by Mr. John Prine! Hey, I know people!

We've been keeping busy with the benefit, in a sense, that we haven't had much time to worry about the surgery that has been rapidly approaching and is now here! We are leaving for the hotel tomorrow about 6 pm. I think that will be a pretty good time to miss traffic, hopefully! My goal is to keep mom as relaxed as possible. Therefore, I think it's a good idea to leave at a casual rate (as she doesn't like to rush) and get checked into the hotel and try to laugh and relax as much as possible before we arrive at Moffitt at 5:15 am Wednesday morning. Mom is being a brave little soldier throughout this whole process. I'm so proud of her!

I'm so glad we're taking little Roxy with us. It will be her first 'vacation'! She's never stayed away from home except when my Grandmother passed away and when mom was getting her port. We had to put her in the kennel and she didn't eat while she was there, so I will just feel better knowing that she will be eating and sleeping with me. I don't want to be stressed about both my girls!!

Joe & Janice took us to dinner Sunday night, along with Lauren and Austin. It was a really nice time. We did a lot of laughing and jabbing fun at one another. That's what we like to do most of all! If it weren't for laughing, you'd do nothing but cry.

Anyway, I have much to do before our several day journey at Moffitt so I better come to a close. I will keep you all updated through the blog of her progress and success as much as I am able. Please say some extra prayers for mom during this process. It all helps. And thanks so much for all your support!! We love you all.

Mom's a CHAMP!! (2009-07-08 23:11) - Beth

We arrived at Moffitt at 5:10; Mom's appointment, 5:15. She's so cute! She hates to be late . . . even for bilateral mastectomies. She was amazingly calm on the outside; although, Jan & I were too, but had huge amounts of emotional turmoil on the inside.

They took her back to pre-op and had her put on one of those 'blow up your skirt' gowns. They're really cool. They actually hook up a hose to the gown and it blows hot air in to keep you warm. And good thing, man they keep those places cold! We should all be allowed the luxury of such a gown.

The players began appearing to introduce themselves. Dr. S came in to tell us the process and answer any final questions. He is so awesome! I had to hug him and tell him to take care of my mother because she's the best there is and I want to keep her around. He assured me he would. Hugging mom for the last time was extremely difficult! I could feel myself tearing up no matter how hard I was trying to fight them off. But I needed to be strong for her and couldn't let her see me cry. My eyes were welling and she was looking me square in the eye. I must have hugged her four times before it was time. I really didn't want them to take her away, but at exactly 7:15 they wheeled her off!

They give the family a number that you can then check a computer screen to follow the processes of your loved one. It indicated that she wouldn't be out of surgery until 10:15 am. At 9 on the dot, Dr. S. was heading towards us. We instantly panicked thinking something was wrong since he was coming out so early. He told us that she did great and it was a 'boring' surgery (which is a good thing). There were no surprises. It didn't look like there was cancer in the left breast but wouldn't know for sure until the pathology reports came back. He had taken both breasts, one lymph node on the left side and fatty tissue on the right side. He won't be sure how many lymph nodes he took on the right side until the final report.

Please keep in mind that I may not be 100 % accurate on this technical information. This is usually the information that my mom fills you in on. Janny & I are so exhausted that it's hard to remember all those details. My specialty is the emotional side.

This . . . I can do.

Mom looks great. She actually looked better than after her port surgery. To see her face, you wouldn't know she just underwent a major surgery. She was, of course, very tired from the drugs, and hurting. We didn't stay too long once she was in her room and we got her situated. I wanted to leave so she could get some rest and not have to worry about entertaining anyone. I told her I'd be back later to check on her.

I went back around 8:30. She was awake and seemed very alert to me, but she said she didn't feel alert. She looked fantastic. Mom said she was having more pain under her right arm than she was on her chest, but they have her chest wrapped and can't really wrap the other area. She said Dr. S had been in to see her around 4:30 and he thought everything looked good. About 50 minutes later a nurse thought she was getting swollen around her port. They called Dr. S and he instructed her to call the resident to come take a look at her so he knew mom's story and could monitor the swelling throughout the night. She told him about the hematoma that occurred during her port and asked if that might be what is happening. He said it could be, but that would be the worst case scenario and would monitor the situation. If it were another hematoma they would have to go back in. After the resident left, she began tearing up with the thought of them having to cut her open AGAIN. I encouraged her by explaining that she had gone through that for her port and it wasn't going to happen again! They were going to keep an eye on that every hour or two.

Mom told me that the nurse had unwrapped her to look at the area and make sure everything looked alright. Mom glanced down and wasn't really concerned (at that point) about the loss of her breasts, but the scars made her nauseous.

Before I left for the night to let my mom get her rest, I spoke with the night nurse and told her I want to be called if anything happens. I asked if that was normal protocol and she said that sometimes the family doesn't know until morning. I told her that I want to know if anything at all happens. She agreed to call me.

I stopped in the chapel and thanked the ones responsible for ridding my mom of cancer and saving her life: God, Gram, Grandpap, Gram Dixon and, of course, Dr. S. Then I rushed to play the lotto thinking this would be a great time to win. Oddly enough, the very first number on the card was '17'. That used to be my favorite number until my mom told me on November 17, 2008, that she had breast cancer. I'm thinking that must be a good sign!

Apparently, all the prayers are working. Please keep them coming for a quick and a not-so-painful recovery! I'll continue to keep you all updated.

Cross 'surgery' off the list! (2009-07-13 10:06) - CJ

Got through the surgery (as we all knew I would), thanks to all the prayers and support from family and friends. The night before, all my brothers called, so I got to talk to all them, as well as Cindy (sister-in-law) and Ashley (niece) and I didn't cry once. I was extremely nervous and anxious to have it over with. Having my 'posse', including little Roxy, there was such a great relief. I knew they were worried and nervous as well, but they hid it pretty well!

After a mostly sleepless night for all of us, we headed to the hospital. Of course, once prep starts, everything happens so quickly that you don't really think much of the nerves. The OR team all came in to introduce themselves, explain the procedure and answer any questions we had. But I felt most safe once I saw Dr. S. - after all, he told me the first time I saw him that he would be with me every step of the way! I asked him if he could tighten up the 'old lady wrinkly skin' on my chest so I could at least have nice cleavage with my 'falsies'. The girls said he chuckled a little and shook his head (as if in disbelief that THIS was what I was worried about), but said he could do that!

I don't remember much after that, including the Recovery Room, till I got to my room. Beth, Janice, Joe G. and Lauren (my little ladybug) came in to see me, bearing flowers and a 'get well' balloon. I vaguely remember 'dismissing' them after a while...I mean telling them they should go get something to eat. I was so tired that I knew I wouldn't be able to stay awake to talk to them. In fact, I don't remember some of the things they told me that I had said.

I slept most of the day, except when someone was poking or prodding, then was up the entire night. I did visit a while with Beth that evening, but it's vague too.

Thursday they got me up and I sat (slept) in a chair most of the day. The woman from Physical Therapy came in to explain the exercises I will have to do for the rest of my life to avoid lymphedema. Apparently, you can get it at any time, even as much as 15 years or more after the surgery. For those of you who aren't familiar with it, surgical removal or obstruction of the lymphatic vessels and nodes and/or radiation therapy causes a blockage of the lymphatic fluid out of the affected area. The lymphatic vessels become overwhelmed and fluid begins to filter out into the surrounding tissue causing swelling. So Lisa showed me the exercises I need to do and walked me around a bit.

In a cancer center, bald heads are the norm, and it's almost as if the patients and families of patients are kindred spirits. We all know what the others are going through and there are always well wishes. And I will say, if you have to be in a cancer center, Moffitt is the place to be.

Friday was homecoming day and we were all glad. Jan spent the night to make us all feel better. Now, not only are the girls my angels, they are also my nurses. I have drains that have to be emptied three times a day and, of course, they are always worried that I might need something to eat or medication or whatever. I honestly don't know what I would do without them!

And in case I haven't told you lately (though I know I have), I love you girls so much and actually DO owe you my life!

Saturday and Sunday were mostly sleeping days. I hadn't actually examined my scar sites thoroughly until Sunday, at which time I did have a little cry, but not a big one. Saturday I only needed two pain pills, but Sunday I needed three. And today I'm already having some pain, so I'm guessing the good stuff they give you in the hospital may be wearing off.

Thursday I have my Herceptin and on 7/22 I see the radiation oncologist and, hopefully, things will progress as they have to this point. I will see Dr. S. in about two weeks to have the drains removed.

Thanks so much to all of you who called and sent text messages and emails to check on us. Please continue to follow the blog for updates and please continue to keep us in your thoughts and prayers!

I'M A SURVIVOR!!! (2009-07-15 10:31) - CJ

At 11:49 a.m. on 7/14/09, I received the best call I could have possibly received...from Dr. S. Pathology shows no cancer on the left side and they got it all on the right side!!! The chemo had shrunk the tumor by 95 %!! He was 'ecstatic' and said that this was exactly what he had envisioned for me! I was already getting choked up on the phone and, as much as I like talking with him, I couldn't wait to hang up so I could really bawl...something I haven't done in quite a while and really needed. Beth and Roxy were coming back to check on me and we met in the hallway, me crying my head off. Of course, she was scared, thinking there was something wrong, and when I told her the good news, we were both in the hallway, crying our heads off! Even little Roxy seemed to know it was good news for a change, dancing around our feet!

More details after I see the doc, but I just wanted to share the good news with all of you who have been so supportive...THANK YOU!!

Glad/Sad (2009-07-19 11:06) - CJ

On Thursday I went for my Herceptin, my first time out since surgery. I was, believe it or not, kind of looking forward to it, even with all the drains and dressings, just so I could tell my good news. Missy, 'the mean nurse', got me set up and was very excited to hear that they got all the cancer. A little later I saw Laura, the nurse who took care of me on the very first day and had told me about her twin daughter having the rare brain tumor as a baby. I was anxious to tell her since her little Sara was instrumental in my 'being brave'. She was, of course, glad to hear it, but something just seemed to be a little off. She said she hesitated to tell me because she knew Sara had been such an inspiration to me, but that Sara's cancer is back. It is not able to be biopsied and she will have her Mediport implanted again next week and begin chemo. She has regular MRI's and in February it didn't show up, but in June it did. If any of you have any extra prayers, this little girl sure can use them!

I am having some pain, not unbearable, but not much fun either. It's pretty frustrating not to be able to do much. You don't realize how many things you do on a daily basis that are 'repetitive actions', something I'm not allowed. I continue to do my exercises faithfully, hoping to avoid lymphedema.

This week I will see the radiation oncologist, as well as Dr. S. for my post-op exam and have the drains removed (which I hear really DOES feel like they tie them to the door and slam it!)

Roxy has appointed herself as a nursing assistant and when Beth empties my drains, she dances around at our feet and licks our toes and when we're done, she goes back to her bench! It's amazing to me how much she seems to really understand that she has to be 'easy' with me. She still hangs out on the couch with me but she's nice and calm and she knows I can't throw the ball, so we play kickball instead! Even now, I can hear her scratching at her mom's bedroom door to get out here to see grammy!

Beth went on a photo walk downtown yesterday with a photography group. I was glad to see her get out and do something she loves, although it didn't go quite the way she had envisioned and the weather was just plain brutally hot! But at least she got away from the situation for a bit. Janice wasn't able to go with us on Thursday because she had work backed up from taking so much time off to be at the surgery, etc. She came over for a bit on Friday but I've gotten used to seeing her lots and I miss my 'seester'! I love you girls!!! As always, thanks for all your prayers and support. I will update after I see the docs this week.

Doc update (2009-07-27 12:05) - CJ

I have to say that the recovery from the mastectomies is the worst part of this so far. The pain seems to be getting worse but I guess that is to be expected with such an invasive surgery. My girls continue to take good care of me, as well as dealing with all the benefit 'stuff'. I know I've said this lots of times but I really don't know what I would do without them! I love you girls!!!

On Wednesday we went to see the Radiation Oncologist, now known as Dr. R.O., just as nice as the rest of my team, I might add. He examined me and explained the radiation process. Next Wednesday I will go for a 'planning' appointment. They will decide exactly how I will lie on the table for the treatments and will mark the areas of my chest for maximum effect of the radiation rays. Once I begin treatments, I will probably have 33, Monday through Friday for six weeks, but the treatment itself only takes about 15 minutes from start to finish. The side effects are minimal...about 10 % increased risk of lymphedema, possibly some burning of the skin (like a sunburn) and fatigue. He says the fatigue usually starts about three weeks into the treatment but goes away a couple weeks after treatment is finished.

On Friday we went to see Dr. S. for a post-op and to have my drains removed. He gave me a huge hug and a copy of the pathology report and said I should have it framed! Of course, I don't understand all the medical terms, but just the fact that the chemo reduced the tumor by 95 % is amazing to me. He was very pleased with the way things are healing on the right side and removed that drain, which, by the way, didn't even hurt one little bit! But in all fairness, that could have been the result of pain pills and Valium! The left side is still draining and seems to have developed another hematoma on that side like it did when I had my port implanted. He feels confident that it will be fine without another surgery and I am feeling confident in his confidence! We will go back next Friday to have it checked and, hopefully, have the drain removed.

So we are now on another roll of appointments...radiation every day, seeing Dr. R.O. once a week, Herceptin and seeing Dr. O. every three weeks and check-ups with Dr. S. I am continuing to do my exercises and my range of motion is good. I will be glad to get back to normal if one can ever be 'normal' again after this experience.

Thanks to all of you for your phone calls. Just know that if you don't get me, I am probably sleeping through the pain. Hopefully, that will be over soon and I will be able to touch base with you. Thanks for all your support!

Things I Have Learned from Cancer (so far) (2009-07-28 20:08) - CJ

...that although I (and everyone who knows us) thought Beth and I couldn't be any closer, we were all wrong. She has taken such good care of me through all this, to the point that I worry about her own health suffering! I love you more than words can say, Bethie!!

...that I love the relationship Janice and I have developed through this journey. We've had our disagreements in the past, as all sisters do, but we are 'grown-ups' now and I promise never to fight with her again! I love you, James!!

...that family and friends are so important in our lives. I'm sure that I would not have gotten this far if it weren't for family and friends, so thank you all for your support and I love you all!

...that pets really do pick up on our moods, and really do help people get through things in their own way. I love you, my little cuddle-bug!

...that it's not 'weak' to ask for help. Sometimes you just HAVE to!

...that everything happens for a reason, even though we may not know what the reason is.

...that you should accept generosity with gratitude. It makes the giver feel good and it's good karma, too!

...that laughter really is the best medicine. Like I told someone many years ago who said 'you can't laugh your way through life' – sometimes that's the ONLY way you can get through it!

...that chemo is not for sissies, but it DOES work!

...that after chemo, the hair on your legs grows back way faster than the hair on your head!

...that there really is such a thing as 'phantom pain'.

...that we are exactly where God wants us to be at any given moment.

...that if God gets us to it, He will get us through it.

2009 August

Long time, no blog! (2009-08-14 17:55) - CJ

It has been brought to our attention that some of you are pinging because we haven't posted in so long. Well, for all you blog-junkies out there, you get a double dose today! (And sorry it has been so long!)

Medically speaking, I went to see Dr. S. one week after the right drain was removed and had the left one removed. Didn't hurt. Everything seems to be coming along nicely; although the last blog hurt Dr. S.'s feelings...he thought I meant the surgery was the worst part! I assured him that the surgery was the easiest part! (LOL!) I had my planning appointment for radiation where they drew all over me with magic markers. Jan said it was too bad they didn't use red so she could call me a redneck, bless her little heart. I have since had eight radiation treatments, 25 to go. They don't hurt, but it's kind of a pain to go Monday through Friday. This past Wednesday they actually tattooed permanent marks around the radiation area. Not sure I could go through that for Beth and Jan...it really hurt and makes me appreciate what they did even more. My skin is a little pink, I'm using aloe on it but apparently, later on, I will need a prescription cream. I seem to be tired all the time and do sleep a lot, but at this point, I'm feeling pretty good.

Okay, now to the good stuff!

When it rains..... (2009-08-14 18:20) - CJ

Beth and Jan have been running their little butts off with this benefit! I have been told more than one time that I am not to do ANYTHING! But I can see how busy they are and really want to help. (Besides, I have been stifling my need to control for quite some time!) Thursday and Friday I was helping out with whatever I could. It was a lot of fun, but at that point, everyone was bone tired. Friday night Beth put a load of laundry in the washer and the toilets started 'glugging' and kind of bubbling up. Next, the toilets started leaking around the seals and the bathtub drains started backing up. Beth and I were trying to figure out what the hell to do...did I say it was storming, thunder, lightning, torrential rain?...when the lights went out...in the whole neighborhood. We gingerly made our way to the flashlight drawer and literally could not see our hands in front of our faces. Thank goodness we had put Roxy in her crate when the water problem arose (arose...get it?) Thankfully, the lights weren't off very long, but still, backed up plumbing and me on antibiotics for a UTI, not a good combination!

Saturday morning dawned bright and sunny and the girls were off to set up. Roxy and I had a nice nap. They did what they could, came home to get cleaned up and back to finish up. Joe G. and James came to pick me up about 4:15 and when we got there, there was a nice crowd, which continued to grow.

Everything looked so nice. They had pink tablecloths and pink and white candles on the tables. There was a table set up with the items (other than gift certificates) for the raffle and the auction, and a table set up with all kinds of hand-outs with information about breast cancer. The buffet was set up on the back bar and there were people walking around with pink containers selling raffle tickets. My niece, Lauren, and her/our friend, Emily, were walking around passing out pink ribbons and free appetizer cards. Beth and Jan had made shirts for all the helpers...white tanks with a pink ribbon outlined in 'bling' for the girls, and white t-shirts for the guys with a pink ribbon outlined in black, and they were absolutely adorable. They even got orders for the shirts at the benefit! They were selling pink wristbands and Jell-O shooters and it was so much fun.

Dr. S. and his adorable wife came and Janice introduced him over the microphone as, 'the man who saved CJ's life'. Someone yelled 'speech' and he stepped up, and with his arm around me, talked about ME being an inspiration...go figure!! Beth, Jan and I were all hugging him and telling his wife how much we love him and she just smiled and said, 'He's great!' She is just every bit as nice as he is!

Several women came up to me and told me that they are breast cancer survivors, probably all of them younger than I, and we shared stories. By the way, Janice's friend, Jana, is also a survivor, but it has now come back and is in her lungs and brain. She is currently in ICU and the chemo is not working. Please say a prayer for her.

My little ladybug, Lauren, had a gift for me, a beautiful bracelet with the pink ribbon and a heart that says, 'Together we can find a cure'. I told her that I would think of her every time I wear it and I will wear it all the time. My niece, Lisa, gave me a beautiful framed print that says, 'Celebrate Hope' with the pink ribbon. Several of the radiation and chemo nurses showed up and it was really nice to see them. I saw people I hadn't seen in a while and met lots of new people. A woman I didn't know told me that she and her friends were going to walk in the Race for the Cure and that they were going to walk for me! How cool is that?!! So anyhow, about 6:00 (how did it get that late?), the sky got black and the clouds started rolling in. People started gathering things up to take inside and it became pretty crowded, pretty fast. Started as a sprinkle and quickly became a monsoon! Poor Lisa, James and Joe G. were trying to hold the tent down and were absolutely soaked!

We think that the rain, starting at that time when a lot of people would be coming out, probably kept some of them away. But it was still a good crowd. The girls had collected so many raffle and auction donations, that at the end, which extended till 10:00 from 8:00, they were giving them away two at a time!

The musicians were great, the food was great, the staff at Ricky's was great, the people were great. It was quite overwhelming to see so many people, some of whom don't even know us, come together and be so kind and so generous!

Beth wasn't able to take photos because she was so busy with so many other things, but Rachel and Lisa each took some. Hopefully, Beth will get them posted soon. Poor thing, she barely got a breather from all that and is now fervently sending out resumes.

To my daughter and to my sister...'thank you' just isn't enough, but I don't know what is. Again, I don't know what I would do without you two. I SO appreciate how hard you both worked and I think you should pat yourselves on the back...you did a GREAT job! I love you girls SO MUCH!! Thanks to all the helpers...Lauren, Emily, Lisa, James, Joe G., Austin, Ashley, Jimmy, Alicia, Tina, Bobby, Buddy, Diana...I hope I haven't forgotten anyone. You're all great and I love you!

To those of you who couldn't be here, we missed you and you missed a great party!! We love you all and, as always, appreciate your support and prayers!

(Jan, ya' know, Beth, Roxy and I kind of got addicted to seeing you so much while you guys were planning this...we don't want that to change!!)

13 Down, 20 to Go! (2009-08-23 21:16) - CJ

Only four more weeks of radiation. It's going pretty well, except that I'm tired all the time. It seems like all I do is sleep, not sure if it's from the radiation...a possible side effect...or just from being stressed. I saw Dr. RO on Friday and he gave me a prescription for a triple antibiotic cream for the scabs that are forming from the radiation, but says everything looks good. I am having a good bit of pain at my scar line and above, as well as under my right arm. I have a little swelling on the left side of my upper chest near my port site. He says he doesn't feel it is anything to be concerned about but will watch it. I also have a little swelling in my right arm and he is referring me to a lymphedema specialist for an evaluation. He says early intervention is a good thing. I continue to do my exercises for range of motion and he says that sometimes you have to 'retrain' the lymphatic system. I am waiting for a phone call to set up an appointment and if I don't hear from them by tomorrow, will call them to get the ball rolling.

Janice's friend, Jana, lost her battle with cancer last night at 10 p.m. She had been transferred to hospice on Thursday and was struggling so hard. She was barely able to talk because of the coughing and vomiting, so at least her suffering is over. She leaves behind her parents, her brother and her 13-year-old daughter, as well as many friends. Please pray for them and for a cure for this horrible disease.

We love you all and, as always, thanks for your prayers and support!

2009 September

And the winner is... (2009-09-12 11:25) - CJ

After careful consideration, I have decided that radiation is the worst part of this journey. I KNOW...this was supposed to be the EASY part! Not so. The itching and burning are bad enough, but the pain that I have often is as bad as it was before the chemo began shrinking the tumor. It feels like someone is stabbing me with hot needles at my scar sites, chest, underarms and (non-existent) boobs! We have gone from Lidocaine jelly to Vicodin to Percocet, which does give me some relief, or at least lets me sleep through the pain. I feel like I am walking in quicksand, it is literally an effort to pick one foot up and put it in front of the other. And they tell me it can last up to several months after radiation. I have two more regular treatments and then five 'boosts', treatment directed specifically at the former tumor site.

Because I am so extremely tired and because I lost five pounds in one week, they had me go for blood work on Thursday, but all was fine, thankfully.

I have had an evaluation and three treatments with the physical therapist for the lymphedema and am now wearing a compression sleeve. The swelling is mild and when I was there on Thursday, had reduced by 1 cm. There is a self-massage routine that I do daily and the touch is so light that you would wonder how it even helps, but apparently, it does.

On Thursday, I have another chemo treatment...my 'safety zone'. The last time I went was like old home week. The woman whose cancer came back in her brain and liver was there and is now doing great! She is actually on maintenance chemo now and has gone back to school two days a week. There was another woman there having chemo and her sister was with her. With Beth, Janice, this woman's sister and all the crazy nurses, it was like a comedy club! Helloowww...people trying to sleep here! Although, with the drugs they give you with the chemo, noise and laughing rarely keep us awake.

As always, thanks for your prayers and support and we love you all.

2009 October

Long Overdue Update (2009-10-06 12:07) – CJ

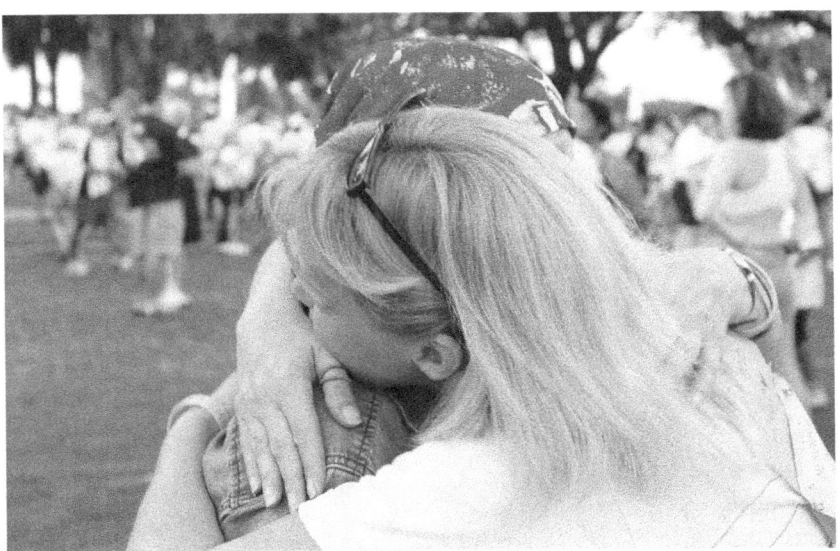

Saturday was the breast cancer Race for the Cure. Janice participated, as always, and Beth and I went to cheer her on. (Of course, we are such dorks that neither of us heard her say to meet her at the finish line, didn't know where the finish line was and didn't even know there WAS a finish line!) We didn't even get to see her cross the finish line and were waiting for her at the curb where the race started until Joe G. came to get us!! Anyhow, she had had blood work done the previous Wednesday; unbeknownst to us (no more secrets) and found out this past Monday that she has mono. So, not only did she finish the race, she finished it with mono!! She is so awesome! Thank you so much, James. I love you more!! YOU are MY hero!! It was amazing, and emotional, to see so many people come together to support this cause. I was particularly impressed with the number of young people who participated and who were so passionate. There were survivors of all ages and senior citizens, as well as parents with small children, who surely had to get up at 3:00 a.m. in order to have everyone ready in time! Hopefully, next year I will be able to participate!

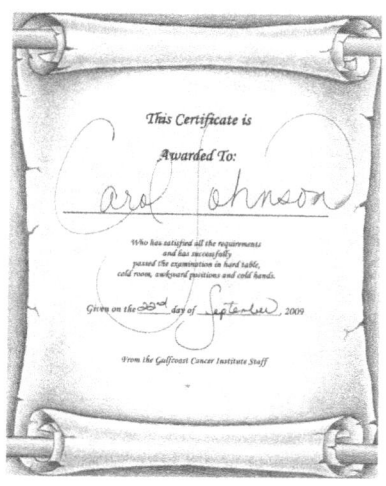

I finished my radiation two weeks ago and followed up with Dr. Radiation Oncologist yesterday. He is surprised by the amount of pain I am having, especially on the left side and thinks I have an infection in my right arm, which is causing so much pain in my chest wall. He gave me antibiotics and Percocet and told me to massage my chest with vitamin E oil. He told me to take a Percocet first because I am to do the massage hard enough to hurt (more). Great, just what I was hoping for. I will see him in two more weeks and if things haven't improved, he will send me for a bone scan. He did mention the 'm' word (metastatic), but I am having positive thoughts that the antibiotics will clear everything up.

I am fatigued most of the time and it is quite depressing. I feel like such a slacker! I just want my body to be able to do the things I need it to do. Unfortunately, Dr. RO says that this will probably last four to six months.

I want to thank our friend, Rich, for the book, "Chicken Soup for the Breast Cancer Survivor's Soul". I read a little each day and it is helpful to me to realize that I'm not the first, nor the last, sadly, to go through these emotions and that I will get through them with the grace of God and the prayers and support of my family and friends.

Thanks, we love you all!

Doc's appointment (2009-10-21 17:25) - CJ

Went to see Dr. RO today for another follow-up. My arm is still a little pink so he gave me another prescription for antibiotics for that and for the UTI I have. Honestly, I wouldn't wish a UTI on my worst enemy!!

The pain in my chest wall is getting worse and becoming more widespread. I am also having bone pain in my legs. He has scheduled me for a PET scan for next Tuesday and will see me again on Wednesday. He says he doesn't think it is a metastatic disease but just wants to be able to rule it out.

He felt some nodules on my left side that weren't there two weeks ago and said they may be scar tissue but wants me to call them to Dr. O's attention when I see him next Thursday. I also have chemo next Thursday, so another week of non-stop doctors' appointments.

I hate to be a whiner but I am really over this!! It seems like every day it is something else!

But on a positive note, Beth, Jan, Roxy and I are having girls' night in tonight and that always puts us all in a good mood...we really are too weird for color tv!!

Much love and thanks to all for your love and support!

The BEST Surgeon in the World!!! (2009-10-25 09:19) - CJ

Dr. S. subscribes to the blog so he always knows when there is a new post. I posted last Wednesday about the nodules Dr. RO found and Thursday morning I got a phone call from Dr. S.'s nurse. She said Dr. S. wanted to see me Thursday or Friday so he could check out the nodules. I already have an appointment with him on November 6, but he was concerned. After some discussion...the nodules are along the scar line, on the non-cancer side, and mostly little bumps, we decided she would pass that information along to him and call me back. She called me back in about five minutes and said that having that information, he felt confident that it was scar tissue and we could wait until my next scheduled appointment.

How many people get this much concern from their doctors? I told Jayne to please pass my thanks on to him, but I want to tell you myself, again, Dr. S., you really are the greatest and we love you! When you told me, way back when, that you would be with me every step of the way, you MEANT it!!

THANK YOU SO MUCH!!!

A Heartfelt Apology! (2009-10-28 07:23) - Beth

I want to start off with a big heartfelt apology. I feel like I let you all down by not keeping up with the blog. It just got to a point where I had nothing positive to say. My mother always taught me . . . 'if you don't have anything nice to say, don't say anything at all!' I've learned to grow up with a positive attitude. Even when things seemed most grim, I told myself . . . 'There is more out there.'

Every time I thought about blogging, there were really negative things happening around here. I didn't want to portray a negative attitude, so . . . I just didn't blog. I am so sorry it's been so long. It seems the harder I try, the tryer I hard.

This has been the most trying times of my life. The day my mother told me she had breast cancer was the day that I felt I, personally, was told I had breast cancer. For those of you that don't know, my mother and I have fought through many challenging times together. Our lives intertwine in ways that some people will never understand.

At the time, I couldn't possibly imagine her doing any of this without me. Immediately following her announcement of having breast cancer, she was adamant that she was not going to have treatment for the disease. I don't regret for one moment that I took the time off work to be at every appointment with her.

The time has come that they are testing her to see if the cancer has spread. She had a PET scan yesterday and we get the results this morning at 8 am. They rushed the test, due to her pain, that they didn't even have anyone to read it. But the radiation oncologist said he would read it.

It's one of those things where you want to know . . . one way or the other. You don't want to hear that it has spread, but you also want to determine 'why all the pain'? Sometimes, you just need answers. Even if it's something you dread hearing.

I pray that it has not taken over her little body since I am the reason she chose to fight it. She has been in pain since being diagnosed, which has been almost a year now. And then if it turns out that it has, in fact, spread and there is nothing really they can do about it . . . well, that would just suck!

Can't dwell on things . . . off to get the results! Just say 'NO'. . . to cancer!!

Thank you, God! (2009-10-28 10:20) - CJ

Beth, Janice and I went to see Dr. R.O. this morning for the PET scan results...ALL GOOD!!! No sign of cancer anywhere! He still doesn't know why I am having so much pain...says I have him stumped. I see Dr. O. tomorrow morning and Dr. S. on 11/6 and hopefully, between the two of them, we will be able to figure this out.

I will see Dr. R.O. in January for a regular three-month follow-up. His parting words to me were 'now go home and grow some hair!'

'Girls' night in' will be an extra special celebration tonight...cheese weenies with done buns and homemade french fries, and maybe a chocolate chip cookie or two!! (A little inside joke!)

Thanks to all Jan's Facebook friends for their prayers...they worked!!

Thanks to all of you who read the blog and support us with good thoughts and prayers! We love you all!!

2009 November

NOW I believe it !! (2009-11-08 16:06) - CJ

Beth, Jan and I went to see Dr. O. for a follow-up on 10/29 and he is pleased with my progress. I will continue to see him every nine weeks while I have my chemo and am scheduled for a routine ECHO on 11/23.

Janice wasn't able to go to our appointment with Dr. S. as she is coming down with a cold and didn't want to pass it on to Beth and me, bless her heart! Beth and I saw Dr. S. on 11/6 and as the title reads...NOW I believe it! He gave me a big hug when he came in and sat and held my hand as we talked. He examined me and all is well. I had a little piece of scab that was just weird so he cut that off, says the nodules are just scar tissue and that the pain in my chest wall is 'pissed-off ribs'(inflammation), for which I will try Motrin or Aleve. (He knows first-hand about pissed-off ribs as he broke one while on a recent vacation. Hope you're feeling better, Dr. S.!) It just doesn't matter what all the other docs tell me, it's not gospel till I hear it from Dr. S.

Feeling better! (2009-11-22 08:31) - CJ

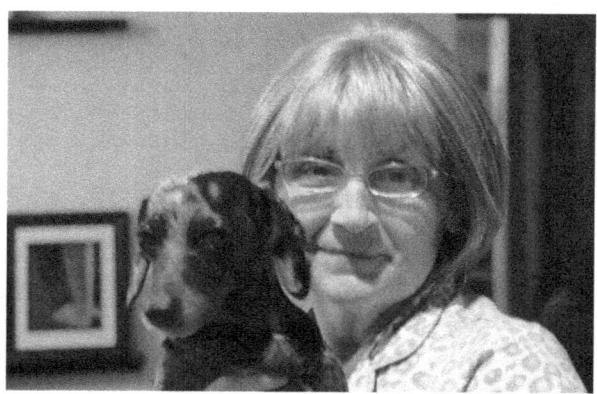

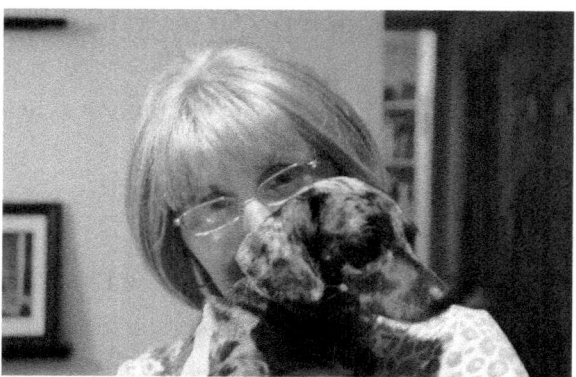

Big hugs to my niece, Lisa, and great-niece, Cassie, for doing the breast walk-in Ocala. Thank you, girls...I love you both!! We tried to post the pic, but ran into technical difficulty!! Can't wait to see you at Thanksgiving!

I am starting to get my energy back, slowly but surely. When I went for chemo on Thursday, several people told me I look like I'm feeling better and most days I am. I still have my moments, but I find that I'm sleeping less, so that's a good thing!

I was having crying spells a couple weeks ago, one particularly bad one, for no obvious reason. Dr. Shrink says it's perfectly normal to feel like that once you're in remission. She says that when you have cancer you know what you have to do...whatever the docs tell you to do, but once you're in remission, YOU have control of your life again and you have to figure out what to do. She says that many of her patients aren't referred to her until they ARE in remission. So now that I know I WILL have a life, I have to figure out how to get on with it!

My hair is starting to grow back in, but it's still shorter than my five-month-old great-niece, Chloe's!! It's coming in very dark, with just a little gray, and looks like it may have a little wave to it, which would be nice after all the perms I've had over the years! (Michelle, these pix are for you...short, blond bob and rotten, little Roxy!)

Beth, my niece, Lauren, her friend (and ours!), Emily and I will volunteer again this Thanksgiving. Beth and I will have dinner with friends, Harry, Rachel, Chris, and Jeff, then go to Janice's in the evening for pie and games. I have SO MUCH to be thankful for this year, though it doesn't seem as if a whole year has passed already. It was one year on November 17th that I told my family about the lump and was certain that last Thanksgiving would be my last.

As always, thanks and much love to all of you for your support and prayers.

I am SO THANKFUL... (2009-11-26 07:33) - CJ

...for being cancer-free...THANK YOU, GOD!

...for my awesome daughter and my wonderful 'seester' who have been so stoic and supportive throughout this past year, who have been there for me no matter what, and without whom, I probably would not be here today.

...for my little Roxy-bug, who was always there when I needed to laugh.

...for my great family and friends who have provided so much love, so many prayers and so much support and encouragement in what I thought was such a dark time of my life.

...for my fantastic team of doctors, nurses and technicians (especially you, Dr. S.!) for the great compassion and care I received.

I have been up since 5 a.m. thinking of all of you and how you have all, each in your own way, helped me get through this last year, and I am sure I will continue to think of all of you for the rest of the day.

I hope you all have a GREAT THANKSGIVING and I hope you all know how very much I love you!

Thank you, Mom! (2009-11-26 09:23) - Beth

I want to thank you mom, for choosing to fight this battle. I know it was a tough road, but you found the strength and YOU DID IT! I love you with all my heart and soul!!

And thank you to those that stuck with us and sent your prayers and well wishes. And thank you to the doctors that didn't give up and kicked cancer's ass!

I love you and wish you all the happiest of Thanksgiving days.

We will soon be running to help offer others a hot meal, a cheerful conversation and hope that life CAN and WILL get better . . . with a little faith in ourselves and in others! Happy Thanksgiving to you all!!

2009 December

Thank you, Bethie! (2009-12-09 20:02) - CJ

Since the Saturday after Thanksgiving, Beth and I have both been battling colds. By this past Sunday, we were starting to force ourselves to feel better and catch up on some things that have been long neglected around here. We did some paperwork, yard work and had a nice dinner. Later in the evening, we sat on Beth's bedroom floor, playing with Roxy, talking, laughing, crying (mostly good tears) and just enjoying each other's company.

I think it may be difficult for most people to understand the relationship she and I have, but it is such a mutual admiration society and it is so special to each of us.

Thank you, baby, I so enjoyed our day and I treasure you more than you know...although you say the same to me!!

You are my heart!!

2010 February

Update: (2010-02-23 21:29) - Beth

I know it has been so long since we've posted, but we've justified by saying that if it wasn't 'cancer' related then it was just . . . journaling.

Not sure if anyone even still follows our blog, but if you do: I have some good news and some not-necessarily-good-but-don't-know-if-it's-bad-yet news.

The not-necessarily-good-but-don't-know-if-it's-bad-yet news is that I have a lump under my left arm. I met with the Ob-Gyn and she ordered a mammo and sonogram, to be on the safe side, given my family history. That appointment is on March 2nd, but I'm not sure when I will get those results.

The good news is that I'm applying for a $250,000 grant from Pepsi for *project: 'I am Beautiful'*. After doing my research, I think I have a pretty good chance of winning this grant and completing this project. Just typing that puts a huge smile on my face. The thought of helping women cope with financially challenging situations while battling cancer . . . priceless!!

I have a very good feeling about this. I can't wait! Wish us luck and stay tuned . . .

2010 March

Thanks, Big Guy!!! (2010-03-03 12:34) - CJ

Beth, Janice and I all went to Beth's mammo and sonogram appointment, 'en masse', as always with anything concerning breast cancer. For those of you who didn't know, Beth found a lump under her left arm and was sent for testing because of family history. All is well, thank God, and it is just a lymph node. She hasn't talked to her doctor yet, but they told her at the testing center that they see nothing to worry about, and you know we all were worried, that is!

So last night's girls' night in was a real celebration!!! Thank you, God, and all of you who still follow the blog for your prayers and support!

Old friends and new boobs (2010-03-07 09:44) - CJ

First of all, I can't believe that I haven't updated y'all in so long! Apologies to all who read it. I hope all of you had a happy holiday season and that 2010 is great for all of us!! Many thanks to Rich, Harry, Rachel, and Chris for your very generous Christmas gifts!! We appreciate it more than you know.

I have had a couple doctors' appointments since I last posted. On December 31, I went to see Dr. O. and he asked if I put Miracle-Grow on my head. He said he wouldn't expect to see this much hair until about a year after my second round of chemo. I told him I went to bed bald one night and woke up looking like a Chia pet! It is still dark (very little gray, thank you, thank you) and curly and is at the stage where it does funky things while I sleep! I get lots of compliments on it and I sure hope it stays curly. I have heard that while most peoples' hair does come back in curly, it usually goes back to what you originally had before the chemo. Other than that, all is well and I will continue to see him every nine weeks.

I had chemo the same day and saw lots of old friends. One man couldn't have his chemo because his blood pressure was too high and another because his blood count was too low. The woman with the three kids was there because they found another tumor on her liver. They had to 'probe' it, which she said was ridiculously painful afterward and they have to go in again to try it from another angle. Her courage is amazing! The little girl who has the rare brain cancer (daughter of one of the nurses) is having a bad time with the chemo, throwing up constantly and getting discouraged. Another woman who had been doing well is now getting around in a wheelchair. It really makes me count my blessings! It's a sad place to be when you hear stories like that, but it's also comforting somehow, that here we are all together with great docs and nurses taking care of us and we become like one big 'family'.

On a lighter note (or maybe heavier), I got my new boobs! Tried on B's and C's, guess which ones I picked? You got it, C's. When I get back down to my fighting weight I'm going to look like Dolly Parton! It's surprising how heavy they are to hold when they are in the bra, but when I have the bra on everything feels very natural. And as we all know, gravity is not our friend, but it ain't touchin' these babies!!

Janice had an appointment for a mammo and sonogram on January 27 and I had an appointment with Dr. R. O. Jan's tests were fine. Thank you, God. Dr. R. O. was pleased with my progress and I will now see him every six months.

Since I started this update, as some of you know, Beth went for a mammo and sonogram because of a lump she found under her left arm. Thank God AGAIN. It is just a lymph node under her arm, her mammo was fine. This whole experience has made the girls more diligent and I, being the control freak that I am, will bug them constantly, of course!!

I went to see Dr. O. again last Thursday and for my chemo. When I went to the desk to sign in, I told Kim, 'I remember the first time I called here to make an appointment. At that time I had decided I was coming only for pain management, not for treatment, and you told me not to worry, that y'all were going to take good care of me and you certainly have!'

Anyhow, Dr. O. told me that the twinges of pain I am feeling are the nerves trying to regenerate themselves and every once in a while, they will 'fire', but it only lasts a minute or so and is certainly bearable. He also told me that I only have one more treatment! I heard lots of excited 'you go, girl' and 'good for you' from the nurses and other patients when Rosie (nurse) announced it in the chemo room. It seems we all like to hear good news even about each other, I guess because it holds hope for all of us. I told them I will miss them and we talked about how it really is a comfort to see each other, as well as the nurses. Of course, I will go back to visit when I have doc appointments. I will see Dr. O. again in three months and from then on, every four months. He scheduled another ECHO after my last chemo just to make sure the Herceptin hasn't done any damage to my heart, which it sometimes does. But I feel confident that all is well.

I see Dr. R.O. and Dr. S. (my personal favorite!!) in May for follow-ups, and I'm sure all will be well.

As for the hair, some woman said to me the other day, 'cute haircut'. She was very surprised when I told her it was just growing back in from chemo. When I came home, I told Beth, 'my hair finally looks like a haircut!!'

Roxy and I have taken a couple walks and I am working out a little and, slowly but surely, getting back to my old self. There are still a lot of things I have to do in moderation because of the lymphedema, or my arm gets swollen and painful.

Looking back, this all seems to have gone so quickly. It's hard to believe that it's been fifteen months. Fifteen months that I may not have had if I had stuck to my original determination not to have treatment. THANK YOU, Beth and Janice, for convincing me that this was the best thing to do!! I love you girls more than you can possibly know. I just told them not long ago on a girls' night in, that if the only reason for all this was to help us forge the bond that we now have, I would gladly do it again.

Beth says that my going through this was her inspiration for *Project: 'I am Beautiful'*. She is bound and determined to get funding for it and I pray every night that happens because I know how passionate she is about it, not to mention that it will be an inspiration, as well as financial help, for many, many women going through breast cancer.

I want to thank all of you who pray for us and support us in our journey. It's great to know that so many people really do care and I love you all. This kinda' sounds like a goodbye note, but it really isn't. We will continue to keep you updated on my health, as well as *project: 'I am Beautiful'*, and we continue to welcome any and all comments.

2010 April

Bad day at Black Rock (2010-04-19 15:55) - CJ

I miss my boobs. I miss cleavage. I miss chemo. I miss feeling good for a whole day. I miss cleaning house the way I used to. I miss wanting to go out and do things. I miss having something to look forward to. I miss joint- and pain-free days. I miss energy. I miss being med-free. I miss motivation to take Roxy for a walk. I miss clean windows. I miss being able to do something for more than two hours without my arm swelling. I miss doing a few errands without having to come home to take a nap. I miss stress-free. I miss feeling helpful and hopeful.

Yes, I know what the answer is...put on your big girl panties and get over it. At least you have family and friends who love and support you, at least you're cancer-free, you're not a young woman with a husband and children who have to deal with it, the house and windows don't HAVE to be sparkling, at least you HAVE an arm, even if it is swollen, maybe you NEED a nap, someday soon you ARE going to feel helpful and hopeful again.

But no matter how many platitudes that little guy on my right shoulder spouts, the little guy on my left shoulder says, he's not the boss of you; you're entitled to be a bitch if you want! So I'm going to give myself permission to be a bitch until tomorrow, and I am not going to apologize for it, and then I am going to put on my big girl panties and get over it.

> RICH (2010-04-24 19:35:42)
> I FEEL MOST OF THOSE FEELINGS AND PAIN TOO – IT'S CALLED GETTING OLD!

2010 May

Doc update (2010-05-07 16:24) - CJ

Beth and I went to see Dr. S. yesterday for a follow-up. Janice couldn't go but sent him a hug, which I gladly delivered! Of course, Beth tattled on me because I didn't call him when I wasn't feeling well.

He called me a 'knucklehead' and gave me a good talking-to! Actually, it was just what I needed (thanks, Doc!), because I woke up this morning feeling refreshed. He said that we are friends and friends call on each other (and told Beth that if it happens again and I don't call him, she should). I told the girls a couple weeks ago that once I got the thumbs-up from Dr. S., I would feel more confident that things are okay...and they are. Some of the things, the joint- and bone-pain and the 'pissed-off' ribs may get better or I may just have to deal with them, but at least I know they are normal. He said it's a balance as far as the energy goes...that I should push myself and that is what I am doing today. Roxy doesn't like it much because there's no grammy-lap to sit on, but she'll get used to it.

So that's it...ten months tomorrow of being cancer-free! Time to get on with my life again. It's hard to believe it's been that long already.

I will see Dr. S. again in six months, Dr. O. in two weeks and Dr. R.O. next month. I continue to see Dr. Shrink every three weeks and will go to her support group the third Wednesday of the month. It is a small group of women, all post-treatment and she thinks it will be helpful for me.

Thank you again, Dr. S.! You have made such a difference in our lives and we so appreciate it. I definitely lucked out when I got you, and your residents are very lucky to be learning bedside manner from you!! And I hope you and your family have a great time today with Mickey!!

As always, thanks to family and friends who continue to pray for us and give us support. We love you all more than you know!

Beth's photography (2010-05-08 15:44) - CJ

Forgot to tell y'all...Dr. S. bought one of Beth's photos of a palm tree the last time we were there. He told us on Thursday that he hung it in his office right by the window, and when he's having a bad day, he sits and looks at it and it makes him feel better! It was really nice to hear that, after all he's done for us, something Beth did can make HIS day better!!

2010 July

Happy, happy.... (2010-07-08 12:04) - CJ

....anniversary to me...one year of being CANCER-FREE!!!

A HUGE THANK YOU to God, to Dr. S. (my personal angel!), to my medical team, to my 'girls', Beth, Janice and little Roxy, and to my family and friends, all of whom knew better than I that I had the strength to travel this journey, for all their prayers and support! There is not ONE of you who did not make a difference along this path and I appreciate you all!!!

Love and prayers to all!

2010 August

Doc Update (2010-08-13 22:06) - CJ

I went to see Dr. O. yesterday for a regular follow-up. Told him I feel good except for the pain in the bones in my left foot. He doesn't feel that it has anything to do with the Femara, erased my fear, or maybe thought that the cancer may have gone to the bones, and recommended a podiatrist. Interestingly enough, cancer doesn't actually go into the bones, but rather, into the bone marrow. As a child, we have bone marrow to the tips of our fingers and toes. As we age, we have less bone marrow, extending only to our shoulders and hips. So, since I have no bone marrow in my feet...no cancer. He scheduled me for an MRI brain scan as a precaution because I have so many headaches. I have that on the 18th and feel confident that all is well.

I went back to the chemo room to have my blood work done. It was good to see the nurses. A new part of the blood work now that I am cancer-free (boy, that sounds good!), is a test for tumor markers. Tumor markers are produced by, as you might imagine, tumor cells. The desirable range is 0 - 38. Any fluctuation or change in marker results are evaluated in combination with physical exam, x-rays and scans to determine the effectiveness of treatment and status of the disease. I will call on Monday to get those results and go back to see him in another three months.

I also saw Dr. R.O. a couple weeks ago for a follow-up and only have to go back 'as needed'. He told me he could see me in another six months if I wanted, but it really isn't necessary. I told him that he's cute and all, but not cute enough to go to the doc's just to go!

Many thanks to all of you who still read this blog. We appreciate your continued prayers and support. Love to all.

Call from Dr. O (2010-08-15 21:21) - Beth

Mom received a call from Dr. O today informing her that her tumor cells were at 47. This is higher than the preferred range. He said he didn't want to scare her by calling on Sunday, but Sunday was his chance to get in the office and review reports. He doesn't think it is anything; however, to be on the safe side, he wants to order another PET scan in addition to her MRI. If those come back fine, they will do another blood test to see if the test just came back wrong.

Mom is acting fine about it and says she feels that it is nothing; however, I really don't know if I believe her. She told me after she went to her last appointment with Dr. O that since she has been having all the foot pain, she was concerned that it had spread to her bones, but didn't want to tell us because she didn't want to 'worry the girls'. So much for no more secrets.

Janny and I are both a little overwhelmed with this new information and I may call Dr. O myself tomorrow to see if I can get some additional information. I am trying to remain positive. Actually, I have just been trying to not think about it today as it is giving me a headache and me worrying is not going to make any difference whatsoever. We won't know anything until after the tests anyway. Sometimes, it's just easier for me to ignore things until I have all the answers and then I will deal with whatever situation I have to. Please continue to pray with us that all is well and that she continues to be cancer-free!!

Love to all!

Round 2: Me - 1, Cancer -2 (2010-08-19 17:01) - CJ

Well, at least I was cancer-free for one year, one month, one week and three days, to the best of my knowledge.

I had my MRI and PET scan on Wednesday and the results were not what the doc expected. Nothing on my brain (hmmm!)...but seems I have a 'rather large' mass on the 'tail' of my pancreas and a smaller one on my liver. These were not present last October when I had my last PET.

Dr. O. says that is rare for breast cancer to go to the pancreas, but that it does happen. He said he would actually prefer it to be breast cancer since there are more drugs to treat breast cancer than pancreatic cancer. He said it would involve more chemo and possibly some surgery (which I have not okayed at this point).

I have decided NOT to google 'pancreatic cancer'...way scarier in print than in person!

I will have an out-patient needle biopsy on Thursday, 8/26, and will see the doc on 8/31 to review the game plan. The girls will both be with me, of course, but I have told them that they have to let me be a 'big girl', going to chemo alone. I know they both feel they should be with me for 'all things cancer', but they both have jobs that they can't afford to lose. I'm okay with all of it for now. We've determined that the first round was fear of the unknown. We know what's coming now so we will just deal with it.

They both think I should call Dr. S. because, as Janice says, 'He's the boss of everything'!! And he really IS...we trust my other docs, but we think he is the absolute last word!! So, Doc, expect a call on Monday! Please continue to read the blog...that seems the best way to transmit information, as well as an outlet for our feelings.

Many thanks for your prayers and support...love to all!

Not Again!!! (2010-08-19 22:40) - Beth

My worst fear came true. The cancer is back. I really thought she was free and clear, but that is not the case. I was so stressed today waiting for Dr. O to call after realizing that we had missed a call from him the day before at 4:15 and he didn't leave a message. That's NEVER a good sign. Had it been good news, he would have left a message indicating that.

This morning at 7:15, I called the Doctor before I woke Ma to leave for work. I have to be there at 8 am but wanted to be here for Ma if it was bad news. The number I called was his other office (the office he had called from on Sunday indicating that her tumor markers were elevated). They informed me that I needed to call his other office today. I woke ma at 7:30 and we tried that office number. Dr. O was not to arrive until 9 am so I went to work . . . reluctantly.

As soon as I arrived, I sent my supervisor an email informing her of what was going on and that if I received bad news I would have to leave as I would be useless. I was rushing through my morning work waiting for the dreaded call. Ma felt confident that it was nothing, but deep down, I knew it was going to be bad news. I could not keep my leg still in anticipation.

By 9:30, I took a break to call Ma to see if she had heard anything. Nothing. She had planned on calling just before 10 am in hopes of catching him in between patients. I couldn't wait! As soon as I hung up from her, I called his office. Of course, he was seeing other patients and I had to leave a message. As I returned to my desk, my legs were barely stable.

My phone rang close to 10 am and it was my mom. She asked if I was inside or outside. I forwarded the calls (or so I thought in my panic to run outside to hear what was going on). Turns out, the cancer had spread to her liver and pancreas. I found that I needed to sit down on the curb to stabilize myself. I told her I would be leaving the office as I wouldn't really be able to function in the office atmosphere after hearing the news. I attempted to get myself together before returning to the office.

Upon returning, I was closing up the projects I was working on and trying to be calm, but I could feel myself welling up with tears again. A co-worker and friend came over (noticing my despair) and asked if everything was okay. He was already aware of the situation. I told him the results and he attempted to console me. I don't do well when people are nice to me during emotional situations so I just needed to speak with my supervisor and let her know that I needed to leave before I completely lost it. I'm big on keeping my feelings to myself and did not want to cause a scene at the office.

I went over to her desk (not much privacy) and she could immediately tell that the results were not good. I tried to speak and tell her that I needed to leave, although, I'm not sure what words actually came out of my mouth. As I began to well up with tears once again, she simply said, 'Just go. Just go home.' And that's what I did.

Mom is being so brave and is ready to tackle this bout of cancer even though it is slightly different than the first round as it is in different locations. I am so proud of her!!

I have yet to have the really good sobbing cry that I need and expect I will have soon. We had a girl's night with Janny tonight which is usually a lot of laughs and we even laugh in the face of cancer. That's what got us through it the last time. However, we have our moments of sadness and emotional drain.

Fortunately, I have worked it out with one of my co-workers that she is going to cover my shift tomorrow and I won't have to worry about all the questions and compassionate support that typically will make me cry. This will give me the opportunity to have several days to get my crying out and then begin to deal with the situation that was dealt to us. I thank her for that!!

Mom is in the middle of a blog with the technical details, but I just wanted to get my feelings out as I found that soothing during the last experience dealing with cancer. I also plan to join a caretaker's support group this time that I feel will be most helpful in knowing that I am not alone!

I suspect that we will be blogging a lot more since it is back again and this is quite the release during traumatic situations.

Thanks for following along and all the prayers!!

The Ultimate Optimist Turns Realist
(2010-08-31 18:47) - Beth

Okay, so I realize that every time you depart from a loved one there is a slight chance you will never see that person again due to car accidents, crime, etc., but the chances of that are pretty slim. I don't know what the actual percentage is; however, how are you supposed to handle the situation when the doctor tells you that the person that is MOST important in your life has a 50 % chance they may survive only one year? What do you do with that information? How do you set aside your sadness when you should take advantage of 'knowing' and make every moment count?

Dr. O told us that it is, in fact, a second primary cancer . . . pancreatic cancer. The prognosis for this type of cancer is not a good one. Without any type of treatment, she will probably not survive 5 months. Survival with chemotherapy, 50 % of those with this type of cancer increases to a year. Fifty percent of those survivors have the chance to survive another year, and so on. You get the idea. Apparently, there is no chance to eradicate pancreatic cancer completely as you can with other cancers such as breast cancer.

How do I kiss her 'Goodnight' every evening not knowing if I will get to wish her 'Good morning' the next day? How do I leave for work every morning not knowing if she will greet me with a hug (as we have done every single day for years) upon my return? How do I go about living a 'NORMAL' life when I hold this knowledge that most people never know.

I've actually heard people say they would want to know when they are going to die so they can live their lives accordingly. However, I'm starting to think that this knowledge isn't a blessing at all. I just feel, at this moment, that I never want to leave her side. I don't want to waste time working or sleeping or doing anything that would keep me from her. I know this is not realistic, but right now . . . I don't know how to handle this!!

The only thing I do know now is that it is even more important for me to find a funder for *project: 'I am Beautiful'* as I want her to be here to know that SHE was the inspiration behind this project that will help so many women and their families! And I can only hope and pray that she is still around upon completion of the project to witness the many people she is personally responsible for helping!!

I love her so much and hope that she is able to become a medical anomaly and kick pancreatic cancer's ass!! I know that she is planning on blogging later to fill you all in on the medical jargon, but I felt the need to let some of my emotions out as I am trying desperately to somewhat keep it together. If anyone is looking for a good investment opportunity, you might buy up some stock in 'Kleenex'.

> Anonymous (2010-09-01 09:31:25)
> Life is a journey. From the time we are born the dying process has started. We are not promised a tomorrow nor should we worry about tomorrow. God's grace is for today. We all should embrace today like there is no tomorrow. Today - serve the ones you love - your Mother. Let your Mother know how beautiful she is right now. Remind her of things that have a special meaning to you when you were little - things you did together. You will have time for the project later. Do things with her now-make things together, take a walk, just let her know how much you love her how much she means to you and yes-She is Beautiful!
> Believe in God and don't waiver. He will get you all through this and know that you are so much stronger than you know.

Art by Beth (2010-09-06 16:57:43)
Thank you for whoever posted this anonymous post. It was nicely written.

We do appreciate each other and the times we've shared each evening with 'The Memory Vase' that I created as a gift to her many years ago. Each night we reach into the vase and pull out several memories that we have shared and re-live them all over again. I guess that would be a great marketing pitch to sell them, huh? But it is true.

However, regarding the project, what you don't understand is that it would allow me to spend more time at home with her if I could get funding for this project. I can work around her Doctor's appointments rather than have to miss them because I have to be somewhere that I make barely enough money to keep a roof over her head. It would involve her as she was the complete inspiration for it and I believe it would motivate her to become a part of the project, thus giving her & I, even more, time together! And for the record, she was told to start a 'bucket list' and she told me that this project is the only thing she'd put in it!!

Thanks again for your feedback. We love to hear from others!!
Much love, to whomever you are!

2010 September

Gotta' take the bad with the good!
(2010-09-01 22:52) - CJ

As all of you who follow the blog know, my doc's appointment was yesterday and the news was disheartening. When Dr. O. walked in, he said he had been completely blindsided with this new information. He said the only time he has ever even seen it was his aunt, 90-something years old, who died from something totally unrelated.

It is another primary cancer, pancreatic. It is about 1-1/2" and is on the 'tail' of my pancreas. There are also two masses on my liver, and Dr. O. says there are probably more, smaller ones, that just didn't show up on the scan. Apparently, surgery is not an option if it has already gone to the liver.

Without treatment, probably about five months. About 50 % of the people who have chemo are alive a year later. There are two different types of chemo that they use. One is called Gemzar and is given once each week for three weeks, then a week off. The other is relatively new and is a combination of four drugs. Three of them are given every two weeks through my port and the other (possible side effects of hair loss and diarrhea) is given through a pump that is attached to my port for the next 48 hours. The following day I go back and they disconnect it. Dr. O. suggests that one and we will start tomorrow. He says that since I am in good health, otherwise (besides that, Mrs. Lincoln, how did you like the play?) and did well with the chemo for the breast cancer, shrinking it significantly...hopefully, this will work as well.

It was a little ironic that we got the news on my Gramma's birthday...she died 34 years ago from breast cancer that had metastasized to her bones.

I haven't talked with Dr. S. yet, but will definitely consider going to Moffitt for a second opinion.

The girls are having a pretty hard time of it, while I, on the other hand, feel quite calm. I have put it in God's hands...His will be done. We have had quite a few girls' nights and sleepovers lately. We just all want to be together and I love and appreciate them SO MUCH!

I have had so much support and so many good wishes and this latest news has brought even more. Mom's church and the church of a friend of Jan's both have prayer chains going for me. I have received so many heartfelt emails and phone calls and I can't tell you how awesome that is!

I am so thankful for all of your prayers and I love you all.

Pancreatic cancer deserves HAZARD PAY!!! (2010-09-02 19:50) - CJ

First chemo treatment today...ALL day! My appointment was at 9:00 and we didn't get out till almost 5:00. I got sick from one of the drugs and threw up several times. Janice said I started getting redder and redder from my chest up to my face. They stopped the meds that were making me sick and gave me two other meds for the sickness. I finally felt less nauseous and someone came in with a take-out container full of something that did not agree with my nose...or my stomach. They moved me over to the other side, where I promptly threw up again. They stopped the meds again and gave me more anti-nausea meds and something to make me sleep. Blessed relief!

Beth wasn't able to go today as she has missed several days of work over this already. Of course, she was devastated. She still wanted to be kept in the loop so Jan and she were texting back and forth, which made her a nervous wreck that she wasn't there...even though she couldn't have done a thing! But my girls are always there for me. I LOVE YOU TWO VERY MUCH AND THANK GOD FOR YOU EVERY NIGHT!!

For the next two days, I will be wearing my fanny-pack filled with another bag of meds being pumped into my port. I will go Saturday morning to have it disconnected. In addition, from 9/4 to 9/20, I will have at least 10 docs' appointments. Five of those days in a row, I will go in for a shot of Neupogen as the chemo drugs lower your blood counts.

The treatment will be a six-month course, every two weeks. They will rearrange my meds next time in order to try to avoid some of the problems of today. One of the really weird side effects is poor tolerance to cold temperatures. I drink mostly only water, and always ice-cold and I can't do that anymore. Today even room temperature water is making my lips and tongue tingle...like the classic Pop Rocks candy. They said cold drinks or food can make you feel like your throat is closing up...it isn't, but it feels like it. Also, touching refrigerated or frozen foods can make your fingers and hands tingle. Yeah, this is a lot more complicated than I thought it would be!

The meds that I am taking (this is mostly a heads-up for you, Dr. S.) are Covorin, Folinic Acid - a type of vitamin, given with chemo either to make the chemo drug more effective or to lessen its side effects.

Camptosar, CPT-11 - hormone antineoplastic agent which slows or stops the growth of cancer cells in the body.

Eloxatin, an alkylating agent which slows or stops the growth of cancer cells in the body.

5FU (quite appropriately named, in my humble opinion!), Fluorouracil - an antimetabolite used to treat cancer of the colon, rectum, breast, pancreas, and stomach. This is the one that is pumping into my port for the next two days.

The most common side effects with these drugs are mouth sores or skin rashes, diarrhea, cramps, numbness and tingling in hands and/or feet from nerve irritation, numbness of lips, decreased white blood cell count with increased risk of infection, decreased platelet count with increased risk of bleeding, poor tolerance to cold temperatures.

Dr. S. called today and said he will get me in up there asap for a second opinion, so I will call tomorrow to set something up.

Hopefully, the next time you hear from me, it will be a little more pleasant news, but like I said yesterday...ya' gotta' take the bad with the good.

Many thanks and love to y'all.

One week down (2010-09-10 13:09) - CJ

I have completed my first week of chemo, Neupogen and blood work. It really sucked! A little reminder...the list of my side effects is not for the faint of heart! Although my blood counts were fine yesterday, I feel like the walking dead. My legs feel like Gumby legs, my headaches almost constantly, I range from constipation to diarrhea, my stomach hurts, I have no appetite and most foods don't agree with me, I'm up at night with dry heaves, I've lost five pounds (I'm not so upset about THAT one!) and I am constantly tired. They tell me the drugs are wicked but they work. Not much consolation at this point.

I have a consult at Moffitt on Monday for a second opinion, although they think I have an excellent oncologist down here. Even though Dr. S. recommended this doc, I just don't think I'll be lucky enough to get another one as compassionate and caring as Dr. S.!

Janice came over last night for girls' night in and that always makes me feel better because we laugh and carry on, and can kind of forget what's going on for a while. Or we make jokes, but most of you probably aren't ready for them yet.

I guess I could put my big-girl panties on and get over it...but I just don't want to! I will let y'all know about Monday's appointment.

Many thanks and love to all!

3 am??? (2010-09-13 20:45) - Beth

As I sit here and type, it feels as though it is 3 am and in reality, it is only 8:45 pm. I have absolutely no energy level anymore at all!

Made the trek to Moffitt in Tampa for the 'second opinion' we were hoping would just be a crazy mix up in the records, or some morbid hidden camera show or anything that would make this all just go away. Basically, turned out to be kind of a wasted trip altogether. Dr. GI was alright as far as personality (couldn't touch Dr. S, of course), but we liked him. He was having a difficult time getting the electronic medical records to pull up from the CD so decided to come in and talk with us while it was uploading.

There sure are a lot of things to think about!! I love my mother with all of my heart! Selfishly, I want her here with me as long as I can and longer. Unselfishly, I love her so much that I don't want her hanging on in pain for the duration of her life. I would rather she enjoy a shorter amount of time than suffer a longer amount of time. That's just our secret for now. Don't tell her I said that yet. I know deep in my heart that I don't want her to suffer, but I really am not ready to think of life without her in it!

I want to hear what all the options are and we are working to get the GI Center the information they need to provide us with that second opinion.

So anyway, Dr. GI goes to check the PET scan records again and comes back with 'I have bad news'. We're thinking he's about to tell us that she has two days left to live. He says that he is unable to pull up her records. I said, 'Never walk into a room saying that when we are hoping for the best, but preparing for the worst!' He did apologize and we all had a little chuckle . . . but it really wasn't THAT funny!!!

That's all I have to report at this time. Just thought I should type something since I haven't for a while and I feel like I'm losing my mind and thought it would be good to release some of the tension. Don't know if it really helped yet, but I suppose it didn't hurt!!

Thanks, much and love to all!!!

'...but you're in such good health, otherwise.' (2010-09-15 09:15) - CJ

The docs keep telling me this but fat lot of good THAT does me! My guess is that this blog will be pretty busy with all these wild emotions flying around!

I had my appointment at Moffitt on Monday for a second opinion. Dr. GI seems nice enough so far...but he's no Dr. S.! I had taken what they asked for as far as medical records, scans, etc. Apparently, he wanted to see the actual slides, so with a flurry of activity to get the additional records, phone calls back and forth and a courier to come pick everything up, it should have been there last night. I think today is the day they all get together to discuss cases, hence the rush to get the slides.

He may want to do a biopsy of the liver to determine if the masses there are breast or pancreatic cancer. In either case, he really didn't sound very positive. He says maybe a year, with or without chemo. Okay, the chemo made me so sick last time, is it worth it to continue for six months? In addition, your body doesn't get used to the chemo as it progresses...it gets worse. Or is it even worse than that without the chemo? If surgery is an option, the recovery time is quite lengthy. Is it worth it? Or is it even worse without the surgery? It's like the commercial...'do you want the heartburn to hurt now or later?'

Of course, I knew from the get-go that the prognosis for this crummy disease was not good, but it is now starting to sink in. Sure, we all have to go someday, but I don't want to leave my posse yet. It's kind of a double-edged sword, knowing that you may have a year left to live, although we all know that we should live each day as though it's our last. And we all know that only God truly knows how much time each of us has before we leave this earth. I find that the calm has turned to somewhat of a panic...what do I do first?

I guess, at this point, my only option is to wait for more information before I can make any decisions. I'm expecting a call from Dr. GI by Friday or I will call him to see if any further information is available. I've got my good, old 'pro/con' sheet ready to go. And maybe I'll clean out a drawer or two.

Thanks and love to all for reading our ranting!

NOW what?? (2010-09-17 15:21) - CJ

Received a call from Dr. GI's office this afternoon to schedule me for another CAT scan, this time my abdomen and pelvis. I think I must have invented some new, crazy kind of cancer, as these things have not been mentioned before. They wanted me to come in on Monday, but that's chemo day and I'm expecting at least a week of feeling poorly if last time was any indication. So instead, I am scheduled for 9/28.

I have a call into his nurse to see if I can get any further information over the phone, or if I could possibly have the CAT down here.

I went for my blood work yesterday and my white count is down so I had a shot of Neupogen and will have another on Saturday. Otherwise, my white count will be too low to have my chemo on Monday. Damn the bad luck, huh?!!

Each day just seems to bring more and more bad news. Better go clean out another drawer. Love to all.

Weekly report (2010-09-24 06:41) - CJ

I spoke with Dr. GI's nurse as well as Dr. GI. The reason for the CT of my abdomen and pelvis is to see if it would be a possibility to biopsy my liver. He wants to be certain that the tumors on my liver are, indeed, pancreatic. I will have the scan down here and they will send him the results.

I saw the doc before chemo on Monday. He said my tumor markers are now in the 2000 range, WAY high!

Of course, Beth and Jan were in constant contact during the chemo by texting because my little girl worries so much about me! They changed my meds around to try to keep the nausea at bay and it worked for a while but I still ended up sick at the end. The meds make me so shaky that I have a hard time walking. They also prescribed additional meds to help with post-chemo nausea and they have helped some so far. They scheduled my CT for Thursday.

Janice and I were the last to leave because it takes all day. 'Missy, the mean nurse' (who, incidentally, lost her husband to cancer when she was only 30, that's how she met Dr. O.) sat with us and talked and answered our questions, some of which were pretty disheartening. At one point, all three of us were crying, but she knew just when and how to get us back to laughing. And, of course, a big hug at the end!! She loves her work and tells it true, and that's the kind of information I need to make my decisions.

Jan stayed with Beth, Roxy and me for a while then left to do her thing. She made the executive decision to come over on Tuesday to give Roxy a break from 'watching' me. It's really cute...when Beth goes to work in the morning, she always tells Roxy to 'watch Grammy'. And that's exactly what she does, when she's not sleeping, that is. She will sit and WATCH me. I told her I do believe she's taking this a little too literally.

Wednesday, back to have my pump removed and home to rest. I am feeling a little better than I did after the first treatment, but still so tired.

Thursday, Janice and I went for the CT scan. Signed in and got my two big bottles of banana junk to drink. Went upstairs for my Neupogen shot and back down for the scan. All went well with that as far as the procedure and they will send the results to Dr. GI.

Today, Saturday and Sunday I go for another Neupogen shot, then Monday for blood work. I should hear from Dr. GI early next week and I will try another dose of chemo, then I may have some tough decisions to make. Not looking forward to it.

The girls and I have been having some pretty real discussions and we have all decided that it is totally necessary for each of us to ask for what we need from the others. I so love and appreciate them. I know how hard this is for them, especially when they have to go on with their regular lives. They arrange their schedules to suit mine, no matter what.

And on top of that, Janice is doing the Alzheimer's walk this Saturday...Go, James!!!

Thanks and love to all, as always, for your prayers and support!

> Art by Beth (2010-09-24 20:15:44)
> I will have you know, that the hardest part is knowing that you won't be there one day . . . not re-arranging our schedules. That's the easy part.

Neupogen Shots (2010-09-28 10:51) - CJ

I went for my Neupogen shots on Saturday and Sunday and blood work on Monday. My counts are down a little and I was feeling so shaky that they gave me a liter of fluids, which did seem to help a little by late afternoon.

Potentially GREAT news!! (2010-09-28 20:48) - Beth

Sorry, it's been so long since I've been in touch. I've kinda had a lot going on lately, but that's no excuse. I have some news. I may be in the running for a $250,000 Pepsi 'Refresh Everything' grant. I will know in two days and I cannot wait. I have been trying to submit this project for eight months and for one reason or another; could not get it submitted. On this day, we got mom's diagnoses of her having a second primary pancreatic cancer, the day of birth of my Great-Grandmother who happened to die of breast cancer and the ninth month after having attempted submission . . . it was accepted without any incidence. Weird, huh?!

Turns out, we will find out we are the winners the 1st of November and could potentially shoot my first hero on the 17th of November, which is when my mother 'confessed' to me that she had breast cancer, as if she had done something wrong. And . . . the day we learn that we are in the running, is the anniversary of my Grandfather's death. All the stars are lining up. I think this is it for us. I choose to believe that because it's all in what you believe, that YOU MAKE HAPPEN. The saddest part is that you cannot defeat death. If only you could . . . think of the possibilities.

Anyway, this is the Press Release that I'm going to submit to the media because I think this makes a great 'Human Interest' story! Would love to hear your thoughts.

Press Release

FOR IMMEDIATE RELEASE

October 1, 2010

CONTACT:

Beth Pauvlinch

727.432.8856

LOCAL WOMAN IN THE RUNNING FOR A QUARTER MILLION DOLLAR GRANT FOR BREAST CANCER PROJECT

St. Petersburg, FL – Beth Pauvlinch, a photographer, artist & St. Petersburg resident is competing for a $250,000 Pepsi-Cola 'Refresh Everything' grant, with which she has decided she would like to pay tribute to breast cancer patients & survivors . . . to empower them with their femininity. She will utilize the grant in creating a Fine Art photography book showcasing these women's' beauty and femininity. Proceeds from sales of the book (potential . . . $4 million plus) will help current patients with non-medical expenses allowing them to heal both physically and spiritually without the added financial struggle.

Beth's passion became clear to her when her mother/best friend was diagnosed with Stage III breast cancer in December 2008. As they sit in the chemotherapy room bi-weekly, along with other patients and their loved ones, the common thread . . . 'the C word' . . . makes friends of all, including the compassionate, caring, and yes, jokester nurses.

You hear others' stories. You tell yours.

It became apparent to Beth that these women, stricken by breast cancer for no seemingly plausible reason, had lots more to worry about than their health. Their mortgage & utilities still needed to be paid. Their children still needed to be fed and clothed. Some of them have no insurance and some have lost their jobs for missing too much work due to doctors' appointments. Cancer is a full-time job!

Now add to this the fact that they have lost their hair and will undergo surgery to remove a most feminine part of their body!

'Many women state that the experience of breast cancer is nearly as bad as losing a child.'

'All that I could do was look at her and say that she was the definition of beauty.'

'All women, no matter how old, no matter how ravaged by cancer, no matter how beat down emotionally, need to realize the beauty they all possess.'

John V. Kiluk, MD

H. Lee Moffitt Cancer Center & Research Institute

As her mother was diagnosed with a second primary cancer on August 31st, pancreatic cancer, a sense of urgency has emerged. After all, she is the inspiration behind the entire idea so she really NEEDS to be here to see it through!!

Beth is also looking for survivors who would like to experience announcing to the world . . .*'I am Beautiful'!* For more information or to comment about *project: 'I am Beautiful'* please visit www.projectIamBeautiful.org.

Thanks for following along on this journey with us! I will post more later as I have a lot of emotions coursing through my veins, but didn't want to confuse the 'Potentially GREAT news'!!

Love to all!

> dltoler1028 (2010-09-28 21:58:16)
> Beth & CJ you both know how I feel along with my family and if there is anyone that deserves this it is YOU! You're right the stars ARE in your favor. Can't wait till Friday to find out.

PS . . . (2010-09-28 21:26) - Beth

I believe *project:* 'I am Beautiful' will offer new hope to my mother. She will meet the strength in these women that I have met while she was sleeping during her chemo.

How do I really feel? (2010-09-29 18:33) - Beth

I feel . . . exhausted, angry, saddened, heartbroken, selfish, selfless, hopeful, inquisitive and exhausted all over again!!!

I feel exhausted when I wake up in the morning, when I get my third soda in the early afternoon, when I come home from work and have so many things to do with all of my 'Do Good' projects, when I sleep all day long and awaken without accomplishing a thing!!

I feel angry because mom was diagnosed with breast cancer and against her better judgment she fought it and SHE won! Now, she has to be diagnosed with a second 'primary' cancer which is apparently very rare! Why?

I feel saddened when I look at my mother, my best friend and see her looking so frail, helpless and hopeless. When I look at her and can see the pain in her eyes.

I feel heartbroken to know that she is slipping from my grasp. That there is nothing I can do to help her . . . to take away the pain . . . to make it all better!

I feel selfish because I can't imagine life without her in it and I don't want to. I love that she is the first person I see every morning and the last person I see each night. I love that we have always kissed & hugged every time we see each other and sometimes not because someone was leaving or coming, but just because. I feel selfless because I don't want her to suffer! If she has to leave me early to avoid pain and suffering then that's what I want for her. That's not what I want for ME, but I want what's best for her!!

I feel hopeful in that when the CAT scan ever does arrive at the right place, they will tell us that there are NO lesions in her liver and her pancreas is operable and won't be very complicated or painful! Sorry, she's my world so I have to be hopeful!

I feel inquisitive about what her options are. Ultimately . . . it is all up to her, but I, as her full-time caregiver, need to know what the options are and what to expect with each one. And mom needs to know that too before she makes a final decision. She's fighting me on this one, but I think I'm going to win. I HAVE to know!!

And after having this many emotions running through me . . . I feel . . . exhausted all over again!

> CJ (2010-09-30 08:20:34)
> Oh, Bethie...you know it's not fair to make your old mom cry this early in the morning! I am SO SORRY you are going through all these crazy emotions, sweetie!! I love you SOOOOO much and could not have wished for a better daughter and friend!!
> Fifteen years ago today...we miss you and love you, Dad! You better have those hunky cheesecakes ready when I get there!!

2010 October

When God closes a door... (2010-10-01 12:56) - CJ

Congratulations to my wonderful, talented daughter for being chosen to participate in the Pepsi grant competition!!!! She is now in the running for a $250,000 grant with which she will complete *'project:* I Am Beautiful', a book of photographs of, and dedicated to, breast cancer survivors, showing them that they are, indeed, beautiful!

Beth has been trying to get her idea submitted since February. Coincidental that the day she was able to submit it was the birthday of my grandmother who died many years ago of breast cancer? Coincidental that the day she was notified that her idea was in the running was the day after the anniversary of my dad's death? Or more likely that our guardian angels are looking after us and this is proof?

This is a voting competition and we are, once again, imploring our family and friends to help, to vote each day for the next month. Please pass this on to everyone you know; one vote can make a difference! (If you're a friend of Janice's, be prepared to be browbeaten daily for your vote...LOVE YOU, JAMES!!)

Beth plans on doing her first photo shoot on November 17, the day in 2008 on which I told her about the lump I had...a way to turn a bad day totally around.

She is so passionate about this, especially since we found out about the pancreatic cancer and I can't wait to see her be able to do the work she loves, as well as to be able to help so many women!

Sweetheart, I love you so much and I am SOOOO proud of you for not giving up, for following your convictions and realizing your dreams! You know what the lady says, 'keep calling them till they tell you to quit!'

Much love and many thanks to you all.

Thanks, girls!! (2010-10-03 15:11) - CJ

Yesterday Janice and Lisa, my niece down from Ocala, did the Susan G. Komen local breast cancer awareness walk, along with a friend of Lisa's from work. Thank you so much girls! YOU ROCK!!

I really had intended to be able to walk this year with them but I wasn't even able to be there as I had to go get a shot. I am also now on antibiotics for a bladder infection due to my counts being low. If cancer doesn't kill me, I guess the cure will.

Anyhow, last night Jan and Lisa came over for a girls' night and we had so much fun. It makes it a little easier not to think so much about what is ahead for me when we are having girls' night. We 'played puzzle'...Lisa is, undoubtedly, the Puzzle Master, and played Mad Gab. Things we used to do when I was growing up and when they were growing up. It brought back a lot of nice memories for all of us which, of course, we shared. I am so lucky to have the devoted family that I have!

A BIG thank you to Beth, Jan, Lisa and Roxy for helping me forget for a few hours! I love you all SO MUCH!!!!!!

Chemo week (2010-10-07 13:09) - CJ

I went for my chemo on Monday, with pretty good results. The way they gave me the meds this time didn't make me sick, and that's always a good thing. I feel sorry for the poor nurses because they just laid off 40 people and they are busier than cats on a marble floor. But they still take the time for a reassuring word or a smile or a hug.

I was down for the count the rest of Monday and all day Tuesday. Tuesday afternoon I got a phone call from Dr. O.'s nurse with some very good news. They had run my tumor marker test again and the results were terrific...CEA was down from 101 to 50.47 and CA199 was down from 2068 to 523!!!! So, the chemo is doing its' thing.

I woke up at 5:00 a.m. Wednesday morning to find that my pump was leaking from somewhere. I was supposed to have it removed at 2:30 p.m. I called the answering service and Dr. O called me back to tell me to go Gulf coast at 7:30 to be disconnected and assessed. It seems that one of the connections may have been a little loose, causing the leakage. He decided we didn't need to hook it back up. I got my Neupogen shot and Dr. O. looked at my port site as it is red and bruised, but all is well.

For the next three days I will go for another shot, then blood work on Monday. Hopefully, I will continue to feel okay. I am about to go in for a nap with little Roxy, who is sitting here 'watching' me, as her mom always tells her to do!

My seester has been up to her shenanigans again...she set up a Facebook page for me and ordered me a whole bunch of friends. I'm pretty sure you have to be under 60 to be on Facebook?!!! But of course, she will have to come over and show me what to do with it. I think she did it so she could spend more time with me...and that works for me!

I hope y'all are voting every day for *project: 'I am Beautiful'*...we really need the votes and the month is rolling by quickly.

Thanks to my friend Bob, who left a very nice message on both Beth's phone and the home phone. Thanks also to Michelle who called the other day...it was great to hear from both of you.

Much love and thanks to all for your continued support and prayers!

Odds and ends (2010-10-09 18:41) - CJ

Okay, all of you who know us to any degree know that we're too twisted for color tv, right? The jokes have already begun. Hope y'all are ready!

Me: I can't wait to fly around Heaven

Beth: Let's hope you're better at flying than walking!

Beth: Janny, do you want to come over for dinner?

Jan: What are you having?

Beth: Liver.

Jan: Okay, as long as it's not pancreas.

I have some really weird side effects from this chemo. One is the tingling in my fingers when I touch something cold or metal. It feels like an electric shock and affects my fingers almost constantly now. The thing is, you don't even realize how many things you touch during the day that are metal or cold...your keys, door handles, something from the fridge, the dog dish. You can't just go around wearing gloves all the time. Worse than that, for me, is not being able to drink or eat anything cold. I always have a huge mug of iced water with me. Today is the fifth day since chemo and I do put a few ice cubes in my tap water to cool it a little but it still makes my lips and tongue 'fizzle' and makes my throat feel like it's closing up. Anyhow, there is a point to this story. Jan and I were talking the other day about DQ's Peanut Buster Parfaits, and I was whining because I can't eat the ice cream.

So Janice came over last night for what started out to be a girls' night in for four and quickly became a 'playing puzzle' night for two. Sorry, Beth and Roxy. Beth gets frustrated with puzzles and Roxy just likes to eat them. We won't do that again. Anyhow, guess what my sister brought me? A Peanut Buster Parfait...without the ice cream!! Y'all need to try it, even if you can have ice cream...it's yummy and hardly any calories! Needless to say, she was my hero, not to mention the talk of Dairy Queen! THANKS, JAN!!! I received a call from Dr. GI's nurse yesterday telling me that Dr. GI wants to do a biopsy of my liver to make sure whether the cells are breast or pancreatic cancer. At this point, with my tumor markers dropping so drastically, I think I am going to wait another two weeks to see what the CT scan shows. I'm not really up for any more surgery right now and need to weigh my options.

Heading to the couch for a little tv, or a little nap, whichever comes first. Thanks for reading and love to all. And don't forget, we enjoy getting your comments too!

Good news (2010-10-12 10:56) - CJ

Yesterday I went for my regularly scheduled blood work. I was telling Missy (the 'mean' nurse) about really bad headaches I have been having lately when I wake up and off and on during the day. I use Aleve and Head-On, sometimes they work, sometimes not. In addition, I have had blurred vision several times and jaw pain. Also, when I feel myself tearing up, the muscles around my eyes tighten up, making me unable to cry and causing really unbearable pain for a few minutes.

She spoke with Dr. O. about it and he ordered a 'stat' MRI of my brain, although I just had one on 8/18. I called Beth and left her a voice-mail because our plan is that I call her or Janice from my appointment if anything out of the ordinary is going on, and headed down to MRI where they quickly squeezed me in. When I came out, who's sitting in the waiting room but my Bethie. She was worried because she thought I sounded scared. (I wasn't...I've had all these tests so many times I could probably do them myself!)

We went back upstairs to get my Neupogen shot and have my port de-accessed. Missy said they could possibly have the results later in the day or today. Janice and Beth decided we should have a girls' night and get in some good laughs...which we did. Thanks as always, my angels!!

No call yesterday, but I got a call this morning from Dr. O.'s nurse saying that the MRI is exactly the same as the last one...nothing there, that is, nothing metastatic. They are not sure what is causing the headaches but suspect the meds. And I'm not sure why Dr. O. has to call with the bad news, but Ellen gets to call when there is good news!

We seem to have finally gotten the right mix and order of drugs because I have had very few symptoms since last Monday.

One of the weird symptoms that I always have gotten after chemo is a raspy, shaky Katharine Hepburn type voice. This time, in addition to that, as Beth, Janice and I were sitting at the island talking, my speech became progressively slurred and I started to lisp. Beth instantly began to panic and wanted to know if my tongue was numb. Janice, on the other hand, started laughing and asked me to sing 'All I Want for Christmas', which, of course, I did. She said she knew that if I was laughing, I wasn't having a stroke! About fifteen minutes later as Jan was leaving, she said, 'Hey, you're not lisping anymore!' So as quickly as it started, it stopped. Dr. O. says that I get some of the weirdest symptoms he has ever heard of!

So back for another shot on Saturday and chemo on Monday...and four whole days in between with no appointments!

Many thanks and love to all for your continued support!

Fond memories (2010-10-22 17:31) - CJ

As I stepped outside this morning I was magically transported back to a day...many days...in my childhood. It was a beautiful day, the sky a gorgeous blue with soft, billowy clouds, birds chirping. It reminded me of a summer day in the little town of New Brighton many years ago and I pictured myself hopping out of bed, hands and face washed, teeth brushed, hair combed, dressed, bed made and ready to run out the door with a piece of toast in hand to meet my friends. We would play hopscotch, ride bikes, play hide & seek till lunchtime. Our moms never minded packing us a picnic lunch to have under the neighbor's 'snowball bush', which also served as a cottage or a cave or a hiding place from the 'stupid' boys, depending on our whim. In the afternoons we might play paper dolls on someone's porch or look for pictures in the clouds or roll down the hill over and over again, just because it was fun. When our dads came home from work, it was supper time, then baths, put on your pj's and catch lightning bugs.

I miss those days and wish them back. No daily doctors' visits, no chemo, no cancer.

I had my fourth chemo treatment last Monday. My fingers are twitching so much that they actually 'jump' off the keys when I try to type. We thought I was going to get through this treatment without getting sick, but we were wrong. This chemo is kicking my butt. I will have a PET scan on Monday to determine if the tumors have shrunk. Hopefully, they have...at least that would make the chemo worth it. Usually, I have one good week after chemo and this wasn't it...so I hope this one coming up is better. Enough doom and gloom. Many, many thanks to Heidi & Andy for the card signed by all the kids! It means so much to know that people are holding good thoughts for me! Please give my 'greats' hugs and smoochies for me and I love y'all.

Many, many thanks to Lisa & her friend, Tere, for the card and 'Survivor' wristband. She did her third walk this weekend, and her peeps, Cassie and Tyler, went with her. Her town has gone all out for Breast Cancer Awareness Month and she has been doing more than her share! We will see you on

Thanksgiving and I'll give my 'greats' hugs and smooches! Love to all of you!!

We are going to Jan's on Sunday for Austin's 21st Bday. It's nice to be around family when I'm feeling down...we're all so warped that you can't help but be in a better mood. It makes me feel good to be around family, and I wish I could see the 'out-of-staters' more often. (Just a LITTLE guilt-trip, guys...SOMEONE has to fill in for Mom!!) So, I guess what I'm trying to say is thank you, family, for all your concern, your support, your prayers...I love y'all.

As I Sit Here . . . (2010-10-27 22:34) - Beth

As I sit here, I ponder 'What would life be like without Mom?' Then I can't think of it anymore cause it makes me hurt inside. It makes my heart break!! I can't imagine life without her; although, I must. She will leave me one day . . . be it now or later. I just wish it to be later, much later! I have so much to show her. She has to believe.

As I sit here, I wonder what will happen when I get a benefactor for *project: 'I am Beautiful?'* This is my true calling, I believe! After all, it says so on my wrist. But will I be able to get over my shyness? Pay no attention to the photographer behind the curtain.

As I sit here, I question whether or not mom is going to continue on with her chemo treatments. They are kicking her butt and she is hanging in regardless, but I worry about how much more she has in her.

As I sit here, I worry. I'm sure I worry about things that I have no control over, but still . . . I worry.

Bless you, all!!!

If I'm doing better why am I feeling worse? (2010-10-28 10:02) - CJ

Dr. O. called with the results of my scan yesterday...they can now only see one spot on my liver, 3/5 of an inch, and the one on my pancreas has decreased in size as well. He says that I am the only one he has on this regimen and if I weren't in such good health otherwise, we would be in trouble. He tells me the torture of the chemo is worth it. But is it? It is kicking my butt on a regular basis, I guess as the stuff accumulates. Joe G. has been wanting to take us out to dinner for weeks and I can't go because everything I eat upsets my stomach. I am constantly tired and feeling guilty about it. I lie down for an hour nap and wake up five hours later. My face itches and my fingers and toes tingle constantly. And if the damn things are shrinking, why am I having pain, more often and more intense than before?

I see Dr. O. on Monday and will address these things with him, but in the meantime, it sucks! Then, of course, I always have chemo to look forward to! I feel like an old person, and I don't really like that feeling! I know his call was good news and I should be thankful, and I am. It's just a bit difficult to feel good when I feel bad.

Thanks and love to all for putting up with me.

2010 November

UNCLE!!! (2010-11-15 21:39) - Beth

I had a rough one the other day. I'm not sure why some days are more difficult than others, but they are. I think this one started the other night when Janny texted me asking if her little Louie was okay. Then Roxy was barking up at the dark sky as if to ward off evil spirits.

There are so many unknown questions. Questions that I have that no one seems to have an answer for . . . I dreaded waking in the morning and taking the walk towards my mother's bedroom door. Since I don't know much about pancreatic cancer, I'm not sure what to expect; therefore, I expect the worst. Is she going to still be alive? Are her organs going to start shutting down? Is this going to be a painful death? I HAVE to embrace this experience in order to get through it. This isn't for sissies, either!

Anyway, I thought I would go to Ma's doctor's appointment today so I can ask these very questions. I was pleased with the answers that I got and feel much better for the immediate future. He said that signs of being close to the end are extreme weight loss, mostly. At this point, they get so weak, they can barely move. BUT, he said it typically wasn't a painful death . . . that is what I have to go with!

It breaks my heart that she gets so violently ill during her chemo and that I cannot be there for her then. It breaks my heart that she has survived breast cancer (which she had no intention of fighting), only to now battle, one of the worst cancers EVER. It's not fair. I know, nobody ever promised me a rose garden . . . but not her! She's been through enough. UNCLE!!!

Just things I think about . . . (2010-11-18 20:18) - Beth

Turns out, Ma didn't have a good day today. She was sick most of it. I can't even imagine the hell she is going through, but when I try . . . I get nauseated! I know I've mentioned this in the past, but it breaks my heart that I cannot be with her when she is getting SO SICK during chemo. Although, it's probably better for her and me cause I'm sure I would get emotional and she needs my strength right now. Yet, I do seem to pull it together when necessary. I seem to get most emotional in the evenings once I get home and find out she's had a particularly rough day.

She got word that her family was trying to come down for Thanksgiving, then just as quickly, that all got turned around and since everyone is struggling financially . . . plans have changed. I know she was disappointed. I know she knows that this is probably the last chance she will get to see everyone. I wish I could afford to bring everyone down so she can say her 'Goodbyes' and introduce 'Crazy CiCi' to those she has yet to meet.

So, three years back, we began donating our time to a church on Thanksgiving to help serve Thanksgiving dinner to wonderful people that otherwise wouldn't have dinner at all. Oddly enough that church is called 'Pilgrim Church' (very fitting). Ma has been very passionate about this offering. This year, little meek, mild-mannered Ma took herself down to Publix to 'encourage' them to donate a cake to 'Pilgrim Church' as it is their 10th anniversary and they agreed. She rocks! She can do what she wants when she puts her mind to it. She's my hero!

I just keep wondering what I am going to do without her. I know that when she passes, she will pass here in this house. She doesn't want to go to Hospice or anyplace like that and I don't blame her. I wouldn't either. Will that make me want to keep the house? Or will it make the memories too clear and make me miss her that much more? I really just don't know.

Just things I think about . . .

I love you, Ma!

AOL XOX

An Emotional Thanksgiving! (2010-11-23 19:37) - Beth

I have a sneaking suspicion that this is going to be a very emotional Thanksgiving for me. There is a huge energy looming over everything. There are a lot of things that I am looking forward to and a lot of emotions that I'm not looking forward to during this holiday.

We will be starting our day by offering our time at the Pilgrim Church to help serve those that gather to give thanks for a wonderful dinner and some social interaction with people that care . . . always emotional for me!

Then, of course, the thoughts . . . Is ma really okay or should she be sitting down now? Is she trying to be stronger than she is really feeling? She got this whole tradition started and now, that brat is bailing!

I am a very rational thinker. I know that it is only a matter of time, after all, we all die and my mom's condition is not to her benefit. In trying to prepare myself, I try to envision life without her. Don't get me wrong, I don't dwell on her demise!

Happy Thanksgiving! (2010-11-25 21:41) - CJ

Thank you, God, for allowing us all to wake up this morning! I hope y'all had a great turkey day and are sufficiently stuffed!

Ours was a great day. I started the day off talking on the phone with two of my oldest and dearest friends, who each thanked me for still being around this Thanksgiving. At noon, we went to the church to serve Thanksgiving dinner to the homeless. It sure makes you forget your own problems, or at least makes them a little lighter. The preacher came up to me at one point and gave me a big hug and a kiss on the cheek and told me that the whole church was praying for me. Several of the women hugged me and offered words of encouragement. If I wasn't on Paxil, I would have been bawling my eyes out!

After that, we went to my seester's for dinner with our Lisa and Tyler from Ocala, nephew Austin from Gainesville, and special guest, Joey P. from PA! Everything was delicious, Janny...THANKS!!!!

After lots of good-hearted ribbing, our age began to catch up with us (or the tryptophan) and we all felt in need of a nap, except the kids, who were overloaded on sugar! Joey P. came home to spend the night with us but he's not feeling well and is getting laryngitis, so the memory talks will have to be put on hold till tomorrow.

Beth and I spent some time in her room playing with Roxy, the maniac! Poor little thing had to be left in her 'spa' all day alone, so she was really tickled to see us and do some serious ball-playing.

I didn't even get a chance to talk with the OK crew or my 'other mother', so will call them tomorrow. For all the family who wasn't here, we missed you lots and hope y'all had a great day.

And now, it is about time for me to go to bed.

Much love and many thanks for your prayers and support.

2010 December

I Ache For Her . . . (2010-12-06 20:58) - Beth

It just breaks my heart to see my mom in this condition. It seems that the last chemo treatment did her in. I told her that it was totally her decision as to when she wanted to take a break from chemo and I would back her all the way. I just need to know what to expect from each decision she makes.

Ma's body is breaking down. She has lost 10 pounds in about three days; her legs can barely carry her to the bathroom where she will sit on the toilet with all orifices erupting. She is not eating anything and barely drinking water. She is starting to look sick. That makes me so sad! I know I am losing her!

She didn't get her shot on Saturday and she didn't go again today to get her blood work. She says she is too tired and when I try to reinforce the benefits of her going (i.e., giving her fluids that will nourish her and giving her shots that will replenish her white blood cells, etc.), then she has been a little short tempered. She is having lots of pain and nobody seems to know why. This 'allegedly' isn't a painful death.

I have to tell you, it takes a lot out of me to type that word ... 'death' while speaking of my mother. Although I know it is a matter of time, I choose to believe that once she's been off the 'cure' for a while, then she will be back to her old self. I really miss my mom!!!

I REALLY miss you, Ma! I wish I could take it all away from you!!

Freeing . . . (2010-12-11 21:25) - Beth

My mother has done a complete 180. Collectively, it was decided that she would stop chemotherapy throughout the holidays and possibly through January too. And when she returns to it, it will be the Gemzar rather than the brutal chemo they were infiltrating her little body with previously.

Gulf Coast called in Hospice the other day. Hospice is typically called in when there is 6 months or less, but you 'can' graduate too! They brought her a bed and she enjoys sleeping in that better than her love seat. I've been telling her that for months and she wouldn't listen to me! I'm guessing she never will.

Anyway, for those that have been concerned for her, she is doing MUCH better now that they pumped her full of fluids and are giving her a break from chemo. I guess it's true . . . the cure is worse than the disease! I am just so grateful that she is able to get up and move about throughout the day and function. She has done a turnaround and I am grateful for it. I really want nothing more right now than to give my mother the best Christmas ever!!

Thank you all for your support!

Ashley (2010-12-12 10:14:55)
I'm so relieved to hear good news! I love you both and she will remain in my prayers. Thanks for the smile =) XOXO

. . . without my Mother! (2010-12-23 23:55) - Beth

I just made our Christmas dinner that my Mother and I have made together for, at least, the last 13 years. Tonight, I made it . . . without my Mother. She went into her room shortly after I came home from work and I haven't seen her since and it's now midnight.

I gotta say, lately, I feel like . . . I've already lost her! That feeling sucks because I am trying to do everything I can to just create the best Christmas EVER for her. If you rationalize, you have to realize that this will probably be, God, I hope I'm wrong, but her last Christmas and I just want it to be the best. That's a little difficult to do when she isn't even present.

As her Daughter/Caregiver, I don't know if she's going through a depression and I should be more adamant about her going out a little more or just moving around! I don't want to push her if she's not ready, but I want to be able to shake her if she needs it. I'm so confused and have no idea where to go from here.

Any advice? Thanks for listening.

John (2010-12-24 07:56:31)
It breaks my heart to think what you BOTH are going through. I can only talk for myself, but I would need a good shaking. Through the trials and tribulations I have had in my life, I have unknowingly fallen into that self-absorbed state and it took someone to "shake the hell" out of me to get me to open my eyes.
Carol has been my inspiration, getting me through a very hard time in my life and it kills me that she is going through all this. I would love to be able to return the favor, but I just don't know how.
You are a wonderful daughter Beth. Hang in there. She has put herself

in God's hands and He will get both of you through this.
If there is anything I can do, you know all you have to do is call. I love you both

...without my Daughter! (2010-12-24 10:03) - CJ

I just read the blog that Beth wrote last night and the dam burst...AGAIN. I couldn't believe I went to take an hour nap about 6:00p and woke up at 12:30a! The kitchen was cleaned up and I could smell noodles and chicken. Needless to say, I was crushed. Beth and I have done this together for years and years and leave it to me to mess up a tradition!

I tried to apologize but I knew it was of no use...she was disappointed beyond words. I tried to keep her from seeing my tears so I had a big old cry once I went to my room.

Although, as much as I hate to say it, maybe this is the start of a new tradition. It is a possibility that I won't be here next Christmas, so now she knows she can carry on the tradition without me physically there, but always in her heart.

I guess one of the reasons I stay in my room so much is in hopes that my Bethie will not think so much of my illness, something I am trying to avoid because it just makes us sadder.

Feels like it's time for some heartfelt conversation between us.

...and Beth, PLEASE, (you are all witnesses to this) the next time you want to talk with me or want my help with something, PLEASE wake me up. I don't care if I've been sleeping for five minutes or six hours, wake me up...and I want a promise on that, okay?

I'll be awake to help with the meatballs this afternoon!!

Love and thanks to all!

Randee (2010-12-28 15:15:09)
CJ...I have been following your story for some time now (don't even know if you remember me from Carnival Printing...but I'll never forget you and Beth!) I just want to say...I admire you and your strength! If there is ever anything I can do for either of you....please let me know. I lost my Ma to Alzheimer in July 2007...it was very hard and I will always miss her! I still have the same email address....feel free to vent if you ever want to! God Bless! Beth...same goes to you! We're only acquaintances but I think of you two often!

2011 January

The Holidays . . . (2011-01-03 22:20) - Beth

Ah yes, bittersweet! I wanted nothing more than to create the best Christmas and New Years that my mother could ever imagine; yet, I came up empty. What do you buy for a woman that is fighting for her life? Where do you take someone that is ill, who is most comfortable at home? What kind of celebration do you throw, when the guest of honor is too exhausted to participate for very long?

I really tried to keep the spirit upbeat, but on the other hand, in my realistic sense, I figured it would be my last Christmas and New Years with her. And my sadness overwhelmed me. As hard as I tried to stay the optimist, the realism was slapping me across the face.

This is without a doubt the most difficult thing I have ever experienced! I can't even imagine the emotions that Ma is dealing with right now. She told me last night that she was scared. I don't really want to go into more detail because I don't know if that was told to me in confidence and I would never want to break that trust. I will let her elaborate if she cares to.

However, I will encourage her to do so because I feel that otherwise, it won't be honest and that is not what this blog is all about.

Ma has been feeling a lot of pain and stopping the chemo hasn't seemed to alleviate it thus far. Dr. O told us that it may take up to two months for all that poison to leave her body and for her to feel better. I've talked with her about her plans. She has an appointment with Dr. O tomorrow and wants him to order the PET scan or CAT scan or whatever test to find out what is going on inside her and upon receiving those results, she will make her decision on how she is going to proceed with treatment. I am so proud of her for taking the bull by the horns and going in 'head to head' with this disease. Once she was determined to fight cancer . . . she went balls to the wall and she deserves a standing ovation for that!

I told her that no matter what her decision was, I would support her 110 %. She said that wasn't really what she wanted to hear. She wanted everyone to 'AGREE' with her decision, but that's not the way it works. I have no idea what I would do if I were in her position right now and that is why I won't agree or disagree with any of her decisions.

I cannot feel what she is feeling . . . emotionally, physically, and spiritually. Honestly . . . a bit of me feels a little envious. She gets to go to heaven where everything is perfect and to see loved ones that she hasn't seen in a very long time. She can still check in on Roxy, Janny & me and know that we are okay. I love her with everything that I have in my heart!!!

I can't seem to stop crying . . .
(2011-01-04 21:49) - Beth

It's not even crying as much as it is sobbing. I am losing my mother. I am losing my best friend. I am losing my life . . . as I know it.

Ma had an appointment with Dr. O today. I wasn't able to make it, but thank God for Janny, who has been rearranging her schedule to make sure she makes it to all her appointments with her. Just a side note: she could use some support right now too! She is going through her own emotions and has to be there for her family and work.

They decided to start the second, less invasive chemo 'Gemzar' which is supposed to be much more delicate (as much as pumping poison into your body to kill a disease can be 'delicate')!

When I arrived home and Roxy woke Grammy to let her know I was here, Ma was like a total zombie. She had no idea where she was, why she was there or what she was even doing there. She was getting angry with me when she was trying to tell me that this same chemo didn't do this to her last night when, in fact, she didn't have chemo last night. I would ask her a simple question such as 'Do you remember when you fed Roxy?' and she would mutter something like 'the crystal that the Lord asked for is on the floor'. I really didn't know whether to laugh or cry . . . I ended up doing both!

She told me that she hugged Dr. O today, which they have never done before. Don't get me wrong, he has been a great doctor and has a wonderful bedside manner, but . . . he's NO Dr. S!!! Speaking of, he called today to find out how Ma was doing. What surgeon does that? He is so one of a kind! Anyway, Dr. O always shakes Mom's hand on his way out and she said she pulled him in and hugged him. I asked her why and she responded, 'I just needed a hug'. (hint...hint, Dr. S. You said you would make a trip here just if she needed a hug! That's what makes you so special. And I thank you for that!)

Anyway, that broke my heart as I was not there to give her that hug that she needed. I have to be honest here, what is it all for? I'm going to speak candidly for a moment and I hope I don't offend anyone, including myself. If she is going to die from this suck-ass disease in the long run, why is she fighting against the tides? I would hate to think that she is doing all of this suffering for me! It pains me to see her suffering! That is what all this crying is about that I can't seem to control much without a little help from some Xanax.

I will hug her as much, as long and as often as she needs or wants me to! I will take off work, I will miss sleep, I will do whatever is necessary to do what I can FOR her and spend as much time WITH her before it is too late!

Platelet Transfusion . . . (2013-08-25 18:39) - Beth

Ma's platelets were 16 the other day when she got her blood work done. They wanted her to come back the next day to check them again and if they were lower, she would need a platelet transfusion. The sounds of that scared the hell out of me. Her count had, in fact, gone down one more point and she needed the transfusion.

I had asked the day before if I could have the day off because this was a new procedure for my mom. She had never gone through this before. Ma assured me that I didn't need to take the day off as it was just another procedure.

My boss is ruthless. She did give me the day off with vacation pay, but not without stopping her mouth before she put her foot in it. I thanked her when it was such short notice and she said "No problem." That's where she should have stopped. Instead, she continued . . . 'Lucky for you it's this week and not a week we're busy.' Really? Are you kidding me? I'm lucky that my mother needs a transfusion this week and not one when we are busy? Why can't she just stop?

I did take the day off. We were at the hospital at 7:30 am. They did her blood work and decided that she did need the transfusion. They sent us to the infusion room. There they took all her information and more blood to do a type and match. They told us to go home and they would call us after they matched the platelets and sent them over . . . in a 'CAB'.

Rumor has it that your platelets go up if you eat eggs. It's just a rumor, but that's where I took Ma. She needed some eggs so I took her to breakfast!

We went back to the hospital to be there for Janny's mammogram at 12:30. As we were turning the corner, the infusion room was calling to let us know to be there at 2 pm.

We are always there for each other where mammos are concerned now.

The nurses aren't as on the ball in the infusion room. One said one thing and the other said another. And nobody did what they said they were supposed to! They were too concerned about the game they were watching to notice that they didn't flush her port before they took the needle out. They had to poke her again and complete the process. This kind of thing frustrates me. She may just be a number to you, but she is my life. Freaking pay attention!!!

It dawned on me . . . (2011-01-26 20:42) - Beth

It dawned on me . . . tonight when I was writing a piece to win yet another grant for yet another project of mine, I always rely on Ma's input when I do this kind of thing. I always check with her before I make any decisions just to make sure she agrees with me and I'm doing the right thing. I'm not going to have that luxury forever and I need to learn to do things on my own.

Don't get me wrong, I've done it before and I'm confident that I am ABLE to do it, but it's really difficult thinking of actually not having her here to bounce ideas off of. She plays a great 'Devil's Advocate'!

I also want to apologize for not keeping you all more in the loop. Ma took a turn for the BETTER a couple weeks ago. She woke up one Thursday morning feeling well rested and having no pain in her abdomen. She felt pretty well for about 10 days until she started having pain again. Although, it's not as bad as it has been prior to her feeling better!

I was delighted when I arrived home from work that Thursday evening to find her on the couch rather than in her room where she has spent most of her time. I was a little concerned that it was God's way of telling me he was going to give me a couple of good days with her before he took her. When I talked to Al (the Social Worker from Hospice) about that, he said that it does happen that way sometimes. Our loved ones can be unresponsive for weeks when all of a sudden, they will be alert, up, eating, conversing . . . and then they take a dive for the worst. But he said it lasted a day, maybe two at the most, but she was going on her 5th day at that point.

I just don't know what to expect from one moment to the next. Including my emotions! I can be really positive and motivated one moment, and the next, be totally discouraged and exhausted for even trying.

One of the biggest issues that I'm having right now is trying to determine if I think I'm going to feel compelled to keep the house because my Ma's spirit will be here or if it will just have too many emotional ties and be too difficult to stay. I'm not one that has ever been afraid of change, in fact, I usually encourage it. I'm entertaining the idea of moving to Santa Fe. It's an artist community and I am craving creative endeavors in my life. So, I have no idea if I'm going to change my situation completely to get through this or if that is considered me running from the truth.

I am just getting through life, one day at a time!!!

Also, I wanted to pay my respects to Cassie's mom that just lost her battle with cancer. God bless her and her family! We love you, Cass!!!

2011 February

And The Nominees Are . . . (2011-02-08 19:42) - Beth

For most SUCK-O-MATIC thing with your mother/best friend having pancreatic cancer . . .

And the nominees go to . . .

Not knowing what the feel of the day is going to be prior to seeing how Ma is feeling: psychically, emotionally and/or spiritually

Platelet transfusions

And finally . . .

Researching cremation services because the Hospice social worker tells you that it's best to have all those details meshed out prior to 'the day'.

Well, it looks as though the panel of judges cannot pick a winner. It's unanimous that it is all equally SUCK-A-MATIC!!!

2011 April

Spending time with family . . .
(2011-04-02 22:49) - Beth

We had a great time hanging with family! It was good to see everyone. Especially Cassie. She has grown up a lot after losing her mother. God bless her! Sometimes you just have to grow up faster than other times. She is so sweet and beautiful. She could totally be a model. We have a bond. I had a great time even though I fell out of the chair. It was the chair . . . it wasn't me! It's too narrow and so am I. Cassie told me I wasn't big enough to be an adult. I couldn't agree more!!

Ma is having a difficult time right now. I never know if it's something I've said or just something she is going through. It seems to be aimed at me, but I try to ask and if she won't share then I avoid it and move on. We might both be a little over-emotional, it comes with the territory. I'm not sure what I am supposed to be doing right now! I go in her room and it doesn't seem like she is happy with me so I leave, but then I feel guilty that I'm not in there with her. Any suggestions would be greatly appreciated!

2011 May

I don't call, I don't write... (2011-05-06 23:19) - CJ

...but good news. I have been off the chemo for a six-week test to try to determine if the pain I'm having is from the chemo or from the cancer. I went to see Dr. O. yesterday and he got me in for a scan, 'asap'. The results today showed no significant change in the tumor on my pancreas and a slight decrease in the size of the ones on my liver! So, even without the chemo, things are good. However, the pain I'm having has gotten worse, so apparently, it's being caused by cancer. I will begin the Gemzar again next week with hopes that it will stop the pain and continue to shrink those suckers away!

It seems the first few days after my last treatment; I felt pretty good and went downhill from there. I was totally fatigued, in pain and with no appetite. Dr. O. says that those two symptoms are most prevalent with pancreatic cancer than any other kind. I have lost quite a bit of weight, so now, in addition to having no boobs, I also have no butt! If I did have an appetite for something, I usually threw up.

If I was able to exert some energy one day, I paid for it for the next three or four. Girls' nights have been pretty non-existent lately and that makes me sad because I really miss them.

So I'm taking this as a 2 x 4 to the forehead by God! Okay, Big Guy...you've got my attention. Apparently, there's something you want me to do. I don't know what it is but I know I can't do it lying in bed, so how about giving me a hint so I can get on with it! Last August the doc gave me two to five months, well, here I am, nine months later and every time he sees me he says if he didn't know I was sick, he wouldn't know I was sick. It's just time for me not to FEEL sick!

Bobby came down from Oklahoma to visit...to talk about old memories and make new ones. And as you can imagine, we did just that. We had lots of laughs and he ended up staying three days longer than he planned! Thanks, honey, it was great to see you and I wish you could have stayed longer!! So does Roxy!!

On Easter, Beth, Janice, Joe G. and I went to the flea market. We hooked up with our friend, Dale, and walked around for a couple hours. It was good to be out among people and it was nice that we got to meet Dale's mom. Later on in the afternoon, we had a little cook-out and Lauren swam.

Thanks to all of you who continue to read this blog, for your support and your prayers! I promise...AGAIN...to try to stay on top of this blog better. We appreciate and love you all!

> Anonymous (2011-06-26 15:57:03)
> And if I may add it was nice that I got to spend time with you and yours on Easter. And my mother was Very tickled that she got to meet you and Beth along with the rest of the family.

2011 June

Wow, a lot has happened . . .
(2011-06-06 18:35) - Beth

It's been quite a long time and we've been busy around here dealing with not only the regular run of the mill 'BS' but a lot of other things, as well! Where do I begin.?

On a recent visit to Dr. O and to get fluids, Ma noticed shortly into it that she felt wet under her left arm. And she was. They stopped the flow of fluids and sent her for a scan to make sure her port was working properly. Apparently, they shoot some dye into your port and scan it and they can see if there are any tears or splits in by the flow of the dye. It was determined by a doctor that read it (not even a technician), 'No, her port was fine.' She went back upstairs to continue her fluids. As they were being pumped into her, one of the nurses that had been on the phone ran to her and stopped the machine. Turns out there is, in fact, a tear in her port and it is no longer usable.

Good news is, she was only getting fluids and not 'Red Devil' as that would have burned her from the inside out had it been leaking as the fluids were. The head nurse was very upset about the entire situation!

Now, time for some feelings . . . this is killing me seeing her like this! It just doesn't seem fair. She fought and won the battle against breast cancer and now she has to deal with this?! It just doesn't seem fair!

She is my whole life! I just want to let you know that although I am not giving up on her, I think that those that have something left to say to her . . . ought to make plans to come down and tell her what you need to. I'm not sure how much fight she has left in her. She is tired and I don't blame her. She's been fighting for quite a long time!

She has three options: she can get chemo through her veins (which will sometimes blow out your veins), she can go under the knife again and have a new port put in (not sure her little frail body can endure that kind of torture), or she can give up the battle and not take any more chemo. She would just be on narcotics to subside her pain while she slipped away. Although this is the most painful for me, I want her life to end in a non-painful way. She has been through pain all of her life. It's just not right!!!

I think I'm rambling now. I have a lot more to say, but I think I am done for the night. If you have anything to say to my Ma, please say it. I know she is listening!!!

Love to you all!!!

All Her Angels . . . (2011-06-26 19:32) - Beth

Three weekends ago, Ma had all her angels in one room. Dr. S came to see Ma as a friend, not doctor/patient. It was so sweet, he brought her flowers. They sat side by side on the couch, holding hands the entire time he was here. He opened the floor to her. Then he said what he had to say . . . telling her what an inspiration she has been to him. She made him a stained glass angel after he healed her of breast cancer and he displays it in his office. He said he thinks of her every time he comes into his office and sees it. She needed to see him and hear his opinion of the situation, regardless that the final decision is hers. He comforted her in a way that Janny & I were unable and I couldn't thank him enough for that! They have a special and unique bond that leads me to believe that he is one of the angels in her life!

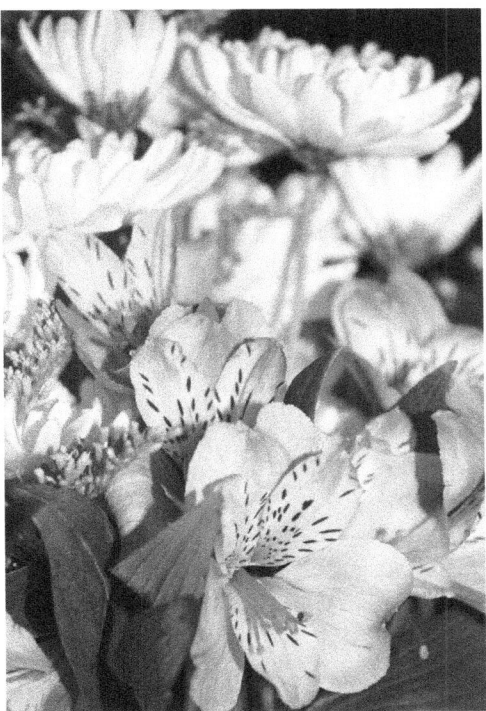

With this, came her decision to cease chemo. She will attempt to live the rest of her days without treatment, but palliative care only. I can't blame her. She's been fighting so long and I thank her for that time! I know that was not easy on her and she is a fighter . . . she's tired! I back her 100 % as do all her loyal supporters. Several of her supporters have been coming to see her and spend precious time with a loved one.

To continue . . .

2011 July

Let's catch up . . . (2011-07-10 17:53) - Beth

I planned to keep blogging each week and make this a three-part series, but I can't keep up. So, here I am to catch you up on what's been going on. The weekend after Dr. S came to see Ma, her best friend came to see her. He was afraid of what to expect. She was better than he had anticipated. They had a great time together and I was glad they had that!

The day after he left, Ma had an episode. She had gotten up and was totally disoriented. She couldn't speak clearly, she couldn't find her mouth to eat some applesauce and she was all around just not with me. I had to call Hospice because I was really worried about her. It turns out that they think that she may have had a slight stroke. The next day, Janny, Ma & I decided that she really shouldn't be alone any longer. They have her on so many narcotics that sometimes she gets really goofy and wobbly. What if she fell or had some weird attack? The following weekend, Janny moved in on an unofficial level. She stays with her during the day and I stay with her during the evening. Then Janny comes back and sleeps here so she can help mom take her medicine. She really doesn't trust anyone with her meds other than Janny. Last weekend, Janny gave her the three Oxycodone that she is now supposed to take every three hours and my mom accidentally took three more ten minutes later. We had to call Hospice then too. We just wanted to make sure she was going to be okay. Turns out, she was.

They upped her dosage of all her pills because my mom's pain is above a 5 on a scale from 1-10. They say that is not managing the pain. We are still working on getting the new med plan underway. It is a little confusing after all this time of having the same schedule, but we will get through it.

Roxy is missing Grammy as she is not really feeling well enough to have her in there with her. She will get used to it, as she has to. As do I. I told her the other night, fighting back the tears, that it is okay for her to go and that we will be fine. I wanted to tell her that last weekend, but couldn't actually say those words. I managed to get them out the other day. It breaks my heart that I am losing her, but I don't want her to suffer either.

I asked Janny if she wanted to be a part of the blog now that she is a semi-roommate and she decided that she would. I asked all parties if they thought I should change the name and make it a new chapter, but they decided it would be best if I didn't and therefore, I won't. I will add her and you can expect comments from her now too.

Welcome, Janny . . . type away!

That's the update. Oh, there are several people planning to come and see her. Her best friend is planning on coming back soon. Also, her brother, John is planning to come down, but he's just not sure yet when.

Thanks to all that support us and continue to read our blog. Ma wanted me to mention that she plans on making some calls, but she never knows when she will feel good enough to make those calls. Please be patient or call her. If you have something to say to her, please don't hesitate. She will get your message even if she doesn't answer. There is no time like the present. Please share with her what you need to!!

2011 August

Not a good Monday! (2011-08-08 10:10) - Beth

This morning I went in to check on Ma as she wasn't doing well last night. She had vomited twice after she literally slept all day. As I was walking closer to her room, I could hear moaning. When I opened her door she was writhing in pain. She kept saying, "I can't. I just can't." I couldn't get out of her what she couldn't do. She just kept repeating it while she tossed herself around her bed moaning, crying and muttering words that didn't make much sense.

Needless to say, I took the day off work. I sat in her room and just watched her. I don't know if I should be in there with her or not. It's tearing my heart apart seeing her this way! She was telling her Grandmother who passed in 1976, "Gramma, please hurry!" Before long she was violently vomiting into a garbage can next to her bed. She says she can't take her pills because her stomach hurts so bad. She hasn't taken them since 4 pm yesterday. She may very well be suffering from withdrawal symptoms as she is on some heavy duty narcotics.

Poor little Roxy was crying to get into her room so she could see Grammy and make sure she was ok. I took her in for a minute so she could give Grammy kisses, but every time I go into Ma's room, she wants to go and cries at the door. There are going to be some big changes around here for sure. Roxy is going to miss her very much and I will probably have to put her on doggy Prozac or something. She's been spending all her days with Grammy since she was a puppy!

She seems to be somewhat still in her room now, so dear God please, give her relief! I wish she were able to just sleep through this pain and suffering!

Janny called Hospice and they are sending her nurse, but she couldn't come until 10:30 or 11. So, I guess we just wait . . .

2011 November

MUCH NEEDED UPDATE
(2011-11-05 08:50) - Beth

Wow, it really has been a long time. I didn't even really complete that last blog. Although, it was quite a whirlwind. Once they came to assess my mom, they immediately ordered continuous care which is 24-hour in-home nursing care. They had to attempt to adjust her meds in order to control the pain and agitation. They were actually here for 3 and 1/2 weeks, which, according to Hospice, is unheard to leave them in here for so long. We all really thought she was on her way into her next journey.

After that, she seemed to rally. Usually, that lasts a day or two, but with Ma, it was 3 months. She is getting very bad and Hospice ordered continuous care once again. I can't imagine God would do this to her again. She's very ready to go! She cries because she doesn't know why he won't just take her now. Janny gave her meds at midnight last night and when she woke up she said, 'Damn, I'm still here.'

She doesn't eat more than once a day anymore if that. She sleeps about 20 hours a day. She weighs 96 pounds. Her balance and strength have diminished drastically. She actually fell the other night twice, yet she still insists on getting up without help! She's extremely depressed. Her communication skills are dwindling away. She's kinda just like a zombie, to tell you the truth. There is not much left of my mother inside her body. It's very heart-wrenching to see her go through all of this! They call this stage, 'literally having a foot in each world'.

I keep telling myself that she is about to take the ride of her life. No more pain tears or sorrow. This is a new beginning for her. I said it before and I'll say it again . . . she's the lucky one!

Gotta run for now, but I promise I will keep you more up to date in the future!!!

Thanks for your support. We appreciate you. Love to all.

Your Re-Birth (2011-11-07 01:07) - Beth

As I sit here waiting for your transition from one world to the other, I think a lot. There are things that I know I've told you before, but I want to remind you of them so you can take them with you into your next world.

For the life of me, I cannot figure out why you think you had no purpose in life! Here are some of the things that **I've** learned from you:

<u>*Unconditional Love*</u>

<u>Caring</u> - you have always cared more for others
then you have for yourself

<u>Loyalty</u> - even to those undeserving

Support - supporting every one of my dreams and aspirations

Motivation - motivating many of my dreams
and I will continue to follow through

Strength - you have battled many demons and still, you survived

Compassion - you cried when you had to fire the lawn guy!

I've even learned from what you call the 'mistakes you've made'. I, however, call them lessons and therefore, I thank you for the 'mistakes you've made'!

You have worn so many hats in my life. You've been my mother, my angel, my best friend, my business partner, my biggest fan, devil's advocate and the list goes on. I know that although you won't be here in the physical form, I am still counting on you to continue being here with me and wearing all those same hats and I believe you will. Wait; can you be 'devil's' advocate . . . in heaven? Better ask them before putting that hat on!! And remember, you and I don't like subtle guidance . . . I'll need it in black & white!!!

You have been the best mother that I could have ever hoped for and I thank you! And if you don't believe that, I know you are my biggest fan so how do you think I became so COOL? . . . YOU!

I am going to miss you terribly! However, I know that you are ready to go and I want that . . . for you. It physically hurts me to see you suffering and I know that there is something so much greater waiting for you. I know that you've been through much hardship in this lifetime, but I am excited for your greater journey that is now approaching . . . your Re-Birth. A place where there is no sorrow or pain. Only joy and laughter, sunshine and rainbows.

The perfect place where everything comes up daisies! Don't forget to water them!!!

In referencing a poem I read from an end of life pamphlet that we received from Hospice, was when the sick parted and we said, 'There she goes.' However, on the other end was a whole group of excited lost loved ones shouting, 'Here she comes!!!'

'The Memory Vase' that I gifted to you so many years ago, it will be an honor being passed down to me upon your departure. And I want to thank you for that gift. I also want to thank you for the wonderful memories that you have shared with me and are contained in The Memory Vase. It will go wherever I may go in my future and I will reach in often to be reminded of those special times with you!

This is how **you've** touched **my** life. Please take this with you when you go because you are my world! I still have many things to accomplish in my lifetime, but I look forward when it will be my turn to join you in eternal bliss. Oh, and let everyone know that I want a mack daddy party when I arrive!

I love you with ALL of my heart and soul!!!

And the process gets uglier . . . (2011-11-11 22:24) - Beth

So, this process really does get worse. I didn't think that could happen because what has already happened has been so painful to so many. Now comes the 'paranoia, refusing meds, forgetting who people are' phase. They call it 'Terminal Restlessness'. I panicked for a moment wondering if that meant because she has a terminal disease or she is actually going to be restless forever! The last three days have been the most brutal of all.

Thursday afternoon she entered the paranoia state. She didn't want anyone touching her, but she is not at all stable on her feet and needs to be held onto at all times. She was fighting to get away from the nurse and me. Some of the things that come out of her mouth are just so unimaginable. While trying to keep her from falling and her fighting me, she came out with, 'Oh, so you don't want me to fall, but you'll let me die.' I know this body really no longer contains much of my mother's spirit, but it is still gut wrenching to imagine that she would think that for even a moment, even in a not so conscious way!

That evening, Joe was here supporting Janny and I and hoping to see my mom. It wasn't until about an hour after he left that my mother lost her mind. She wanted out of this house. She refused her meds, but grabbed them up and wouldn't let go. She ended up throwing them. She was trying to get out of the garage door and was kicking it and yelling. She just went bonkers! Janny called Joe sobbing asking him to come back. He came back and walked around with her for hours and hugging and holding her. He seems to calm her down. After being up until about 3 am that night, fighting my mother's paranoid state, the next morning she woke at 5 am coming into the room where Janny, Roxy and I were sleeping. She whipped the covers off of Janny and ordered her to get up, get dressed and get out. Then she proceeded to bitch me out saying, 'you need to get up and get this place cleaned up. Do you know what your mother would say if she saw this pigsty? You have clothes piled up all over the place and porch rails and if you don't have it cleaned up in five minutes, I'm calling the police.' She had no idea I was her daughter or what she was saying.

We finally got her asleep at about 3:30 pm. Then she woke again at 5:30 in a sad state. She didn't think she lived here and wanted to go home. She walked with the nurse and me in tow all over this house as she was trying to get out. She told the nurse to have compassion as a mother. She said if she didn't get home, her daughter would be so worried about her. I tried to tell her that I was her daughter and that I was very worried about her, but she didn't know who I was, and told me I was a 'lying bitch'. She wanted to call the police again because she is so paranoid that we are all against her. She picked up a vase and was going to throw it through the window to get out. She fought both, the nurse and I to pry it from her hands. Then she took my hand and was banging it against the door. She told the nurse she wanted to hurt me because I wouldn't take her to her daughter. At one point, I had my hands around her waist as she attempted to walk and she grabbed my pinky fingers with each of her fists and was pulling them back and told the nurse she was trying to break them. I tried everything I could think of . . . even showing her my driver's license ('Oh, like no one has ever lied to the government,' she said). We had to call for backup from Hospice.

This morning I heard her over the monitor arguing with the morning nurse at 8 am. Great . . . it's starting already! Gonna be a long day and a long day it has been so far and it's only 6:10. She is finally sleeping, but not without a significant battle. Again, she didn't believe she lived here and wanted to go home. She was refusing her meds. It took us two hours of constant nagging to finally get her to take 75 % of **one** of her meds. Today, according to her, I was a psycho bitch and she told Janny she f'ing hated her. She pulled a wooden mask off the wall that I bought while in Jamaica and was going to slam it through the French doors to get out. It literally took three of us: me holding her up and Janny & the nurse to pry it from her hands. She has amazing strength in that 90-pound body. Then she was pathetically yelling 'help' out one of the bathroom windows with her teeny tiny voice. It was so . . . I can't even think of a word to describe it. The entire situation just rips me apart. I literally feel like I am dying inside!

Poor Roxy doesn't know what the hell is going on and is scared to pieces. When Grammy is freaking out Roxy cries and jumps on her and licks her. She's really been a good girl considering what is going on around here. Nurses and more nurses, outbursts of yelling and tears, mom's combativeness. The primary weekend nurse has to stop by on the weekends to assess. They mentioned respite care. I have an issue with that because Janny & I promised her we would keep her home and not put her in a hospital. She wants to die here. SO, they are going to try the subcutaneous method of giving her meds since she is fighting and spitting it out. Therefore, we are going to go that route before placing her in Woodside. Janny and I just can't keep doing this if she is going to continue to be combative. We are getting about 2-3 hours of sleep a night and it's killing us. Not to mention, it is becoming no longer safe for her here.

Anyway, that's the current update. Don't really know if I got it all straight on the days, but it gets a little confusing when it goes on for this long. We are hanging in, but I really don't know how much longer we are going to be able to.

Thanks for all your support and love to all!

Terminal Restlessness Over . . .
(2011-11-13 12:52) - Beth

. . . I think. We didn't have a midnight nurse last night, so Janny sat up with her until 5 and I went in after that.

Fortunately, we were able to give her meds to her while she slept so we didn't have a battle. She was in such a deep sleep, we stuck the syringe on the inside of her cheeks and let it absorb.

She woke shortly before 8 am. She asked me not to be another one who is going to put her to bed again. She said five of them put her to bed. I told her I was not going to do that as she is already in bed! She asked how long we've lived in the house. She said when she recently went to look at houses, they didn't . . . (she paused). I continued, 'come with nurses'? She giggled and said, 'Yeah'. I told her that this one didn't either, but we specially ordered them for her because she was so special!

Sunday 11:00 am

She took her meds without any problems. She wanted to get up and go to the bathroom, but apparently, her legs weren't working and she agreed to use the bedside toilet. She had mentioned to me earlier that her body hurt and she didn't know if she would be able to get out of bed. I told her I would give her a massage when she woke up some and she thinks she would like that.

Sunday 7:00 pm

We had a good day. She slept a lot and then she got up and ate a little bit of everything that I brought home. I guided her to her room and she was watching my feet. She had forgotten how to walk! She got almost there and said she couldn't continue because her neck was tired looking down. I held her and the nurse retrieved the wheelchair.

I asked if she wanted that massage that I promised her earlier. She sat and enjoyed most of her massage until she 'snapped', grabbed my hands and held me captive for about 30 minutes. I didn't want to escape since she was calm and just holding me hostage. She was sitting and she was safe! She wasn't trying to slam anything through the window. I was sitting on a hardwood floor, but it was still better than the alternative!

She apparently, slapped Janny tonight; trying two more times after that, but missed. The nurses seem to think that the cancer has spread to her brain because she is just . . . I think they called it 'Medically Psychotic' or something like that.

Monday 4:30 am

I was awakened by my mother fighting with the nurse. We decided when we could no longer control her that it was safer for her to go into a facility that they will have more control than the single nurse watching and fighting her at home. This is the toughest decision I have ever made. I am her Health Care Surrogate. It broke my heart to make that decision since I promised her I would keep her home. At 1 pm, we had her transported to Hospice Woodside.

When the transporters arrived, she asked what they wanted her to do. They told her they were going to place her on the gurney and take her out. As I was watching, my eyes filled with tears and I was about to break down. Al was watching from across the room and came to put his arm around me to offer support. I NEVER make a promise that I'm not 100% sure I can keep. I promised her that I would allow her to die at home because that was her request. She just really was no longer safe in that environment. After arriving at Hospice, I determined that she thought she was just going to a doctor's appointment and wanted to go home after she saw the doctor, but she had to stay.

Tuesday 1:00 pm

I was stalling to go see my ma tonight because I wasn't sure if she was going to be upset with me for taking her away from her home; even though she didn't even know she had been at home. Once I arrived at the hospital, she attempted to escape several times, several times setting off the alarm. Then she had her mouth open and was raising her knee to her mouth before she said that she couldn't even eat that. I told her I hoped that she hadn't as it was her knee.

This process is brutal and, really, unnecessary! Can't you just please take her before she loses all of her pride? I love her so much and really don't want to see her go through this!

Tuesday 7:00 pm

I am not only losing a mother, but I am losing a best friend, as well. This isn't fair! I am losing two people in one. I took Roxy with me hoping that would distract her from being pissed at me. Ma is so out of it that I don't think she even realized that Roxy was there.

Upon arriving home, I laid the rose upon her pillow that has a sweet smell and has for months. I'm guessing when the flower loses its scent, she will have passed. I had a good battle with the punching bag. Then I had a good battle with everything else I am dealing with.

I feel really guilty because I told her I would be back, but I can't go back right now. It's too heart-breaking!!!! I will go back tomorrow. I love her with all my heart!!!

Now What? (2011-11-18 21:05) - Beth

So Ma has been in the Hospice Care facility for five days now. Janny officially moved out yesterday. It's just me and Roxy. It's been about seven years since I've lived alone. The house seems so much bigger now . . . and a little empty! It took me several hours to even walk back to that end of the house when I arrived back home. Not sure why really.

She hasn't passed, but we're not sure if she will be coming back home . . . or not. I don't really know what I am supposed to be doing now. I can't really move on yet because it's not over. I feel we are just waiting for her to die. That is such an incredibly helpless feeling. Truth be told, that is exactly what we are doing. We know she is not going to get better, so it's this waiting game of when the actual end will be.

I am being 'forced' into many changes in my life. Those that know us, know the relationship that my mother and I have had all these years. I'm trying to make personal changes for this new chapter in my life. I don't want life to be the only predictor of my life. I want to make my life happen! And I have to look forward to this if I'm going to survive. I want to start into this with my relentless, ultimate optimistic attitude that I have carried with me all my life . . . there always has to be something more, something better! I have a lot to offer to this world and I'm ready to start making that happen.

I'm hoping this isn't an indication that I'm going to AVOID dealing with my mother's death. I'm trying to approach it as I could easily dive into a deep depression over losing her and I want to avoid THAT from happening. Therefore, I am attempting to look into my future as another era. A new life for me to try new things and explore the many opportunities that are out there to make a difference. And of course, I will do it all in her memory. This disease and her strength have both just floored me. I've never been this close to death with someone that I love more than life. It has been very eye-opening. I'm a little bittersweet about people, such as Hospice staff, thanking me for taking care of her. It's very rewarding to hear because until you've been through it . . . you really have no idea the strain it puts on all parts of your life. Then I think, why would you thank me? I'm only doing what I need to do. But as I understand it, many people don't take care of their loved ones as Janny and I have.

Here's to another day!

Unresponsive (2011-11-19 19:45) - Beth

Ma has been unresponsive today which is one of the indications that she's reaching the end. I thought 'unresponsive' meant almost comatose. Unbeknownst to me, that is not the case. She would open her eyes when the nurses or aides were doing something with her, but she said nothing all day! They are giving her meds to control her natural fluids in her mouth. Apparently, at this stage, they really can't swallow and those fluids just run back in their throats, basically choking them. She started choking twice tonight. Scared the hell out of me.

We asked what her blood pressure was today and they said it was so low they couldn't get a reading. Another thing I learned. I thought if they couldn't read your blood pressure that meant you were already gone. The nurses say her demise will probably be tomorrow or maybe Monday. I mean, this is what we've been wanting for her, but somehow the closer it gets . . . the more painful it is. To watch the person you love most in this world just crumble into this crippling body, not being able to do anything but allow those around you to do what they wish and not able to have a voice, it's brutal! I can't really even begin to describe it properly. Why can't they take their pride with them? One of the questions I will ask God upon arriving in heaven myself.

I took Roxy today so she could see Grammy one more time. Roxy is very sad. I'm not sure she knows exactly what is going on, but she knows that Grammy is sick. As soon as we arrived in her room, Roxy was crying and jumping up to her bed. I put her in bed with her and she just kissed and kissed Grammy. The nurses came in to turn ma and she was moaning while being moved. I don't know how she can feel any pain with the amount of pain meds they have pumping into her. Anyway, Roxy cried because she heard Grammy moaning. Roxy became very close to my mother through the years. Roxy nursed my mom back to health during her breast cancer. She would lay in bed with her all day while I was at work. I would tell her to 'keep an eye on Grammy while I'm gone'. One day my mom asked me not to tell her that anymore because every time she would look at Roxy, she would be just staring at her. She said she thought Roxy was taking it too literally!

All I can say at this point is I hope that this is the most difficult thing I will ever have to deal with in my life because I really don't think I could handle anything worse than this!

Go fly with the other angels and eat your strawberries and peanut butter fudge!

I LOVE YOU MY SWEET MOTHER WITH ALL OF MY HEART AND SOUL!!!

Spread your wings and fly, my angel! (2011-11-20 18:32) - Beth

11/20/2011 at 11:06 am, my mother took her final breath. It was obviously very sad, but that is a precious moment that I will hold with me for the rest of my days. How profound that she was there when I took my first breath and I was there when she took her last! Finally, she is at peace. Her Re-Birth is exactly 3 years and 3 days since she told me she had breast cancer.

Grieving . . . (2011-11-21 17:57) - Beth

It seems that everyone wants me to grieve. 'You have to take time to grieve, Beth!' That's what they say. Quite frankly, I'm tired of grieving. I've been grieving for the past three years.

I grieved when my mother was diagnosed with Cancer . . . again

I grieved every time I saw my mother cry

I grieved when my mother didn't know who I was

I grieved when my mother no longer 'remembered' how to walk

I grieved every time I saw my mother get violent (that wasn't who she was!)

I grieved when I was no longer able to keep my mother safe at home

I grieved when I walked into my mother's room and heard her choking on secretions because she was no longer able swallow

I grieved when she took her very last breath of life

Isn't that enough grieving? Besides, I don't like to be sad. I want to be happy again. I no longer allow this vicious disease to continue to control my life and my emotions. My mother claimed her freedom from cancer when she took that last breath. I applaud her! She was a soldier of strength and she fought this battle. But when enough was enough, she stopped fighting. Does that make her the loser . . . not a chance. It makes her the winner because cancer can no longer touch her. Way to go, Ma. I'm going to follow in your footsteps and stop fighting cancer also. It cannot control my life anymore. I refuse to allow it.

A wise cat once said . . . *'Don't cry because it's over. Smile because it happened.'*

Seriously . . . (2011-11-29 21:01) - Beth

I expected a lot more from those closest to me. Let me apologize in advance, but I would think that I could expect a lot more from you. You, I thought, were my closest friends, but I couldn't feel more separated from you. Both of you! I am disappointed in your response or, your lack of! I can't even think that you would abandon me during this process. You are the only two that I've ever known to never have a lack of words. You disappoint me! I feel neglected by you both!!!

2011 December

Ma's Remains . . . (2011-12-01 17:55) - Beth

Today was the day we were to pick up her remains. Janny told me she would go with me. Dale and Al also told me they would go. I was glad that Janny went. We got there 45 minutes before our scheduled appointment. As we were walking in we noticed on the pavement you could see the shadow of the smoke coming out of the incinerator. It was kind of eerie! We gave each other the 'that's creepy' look.

As we walk in, we are greeted by a pleasant man wearing shorts and flip-flops (typical business attire in Florida). I told him I was there to pick up Carol Johnson. Again, Janny and I exchanged a glance as that was quite weird to be saying. He went to the back and presented us with a white cardboard box about the size of a breadbox. He gave us the death certificates and explained that there was a long and a short certificate. Apparently, in the state of Florida, the only people entitled to know the cause of death are those distributing benefits for death (e.g., insurance companies). Anyone else is only entitled to the certificate without the cause of death. All news to me.

I proceed to ask about urns. He briefly showed me his minimal, but impressive collection. He said it depended on what we planned to do with the ashes. Some people scatter most and keep a very small amount. Some sprinkle a little but keep the larger portion. Then he began telling us that one woman created a di- solvable ship to which she could be placed in and sent out to sea. Eventually, the ship would dissolve and her ashes would then be released. I thought that was a pretty cool idea. Janny said she saw where you fill a balloon with the ashes and once it reaches a certain altitude, it would burst and the ashes would be released. Great, now I have to get even more creative with my ideas for her remains. I didn't realize you could be so creative with remains. I mean, I am an artist and I should probably come up with a new project to work on since I don't have anything else going on . . . Haaaa. But those that know me, know I will.

Of course, again to keep from crying as we Pauvlinchs' do, we began with the jokes. Janny said, 'Louie, you should really think outside the box.' I know we are probably not right in the head, but this is how my family has gotten through the difficult times. I'm serious about living by . . . you gotta laugh to keep from crying! After picking Ma up, we went to donate her clothes to Hospice Thrift Shop. They thanked me for the donation and I thanked them for taking such great care of my mother when she was ill. When I got back in the car, Janny said, 'You should have said, 'Do you want to meet her? She's right here." She isn't right, that girl.

By the time we arrived at Janny's, she decided she wanted to see the remains. I told her to open it. Funny thing is . . . we are too dumb to open it. We are both looking all around this plastic box with no idea. We told my ma she was stuck in there! I called the crematory before they closed to find out. Oh . . . this thing should come with directions. Never mind, we will wait.

So after I get home and, of course, welcome her back home, I got little Roxy. When I showed her the box, she sniffed and sniffed and then kissed me. I'm not sure if dogs noses are THAT strong or not, but it seemed that she knew it was 'Grammy'. Time for a cocktail, a Xanax and a nap! Exhausted.

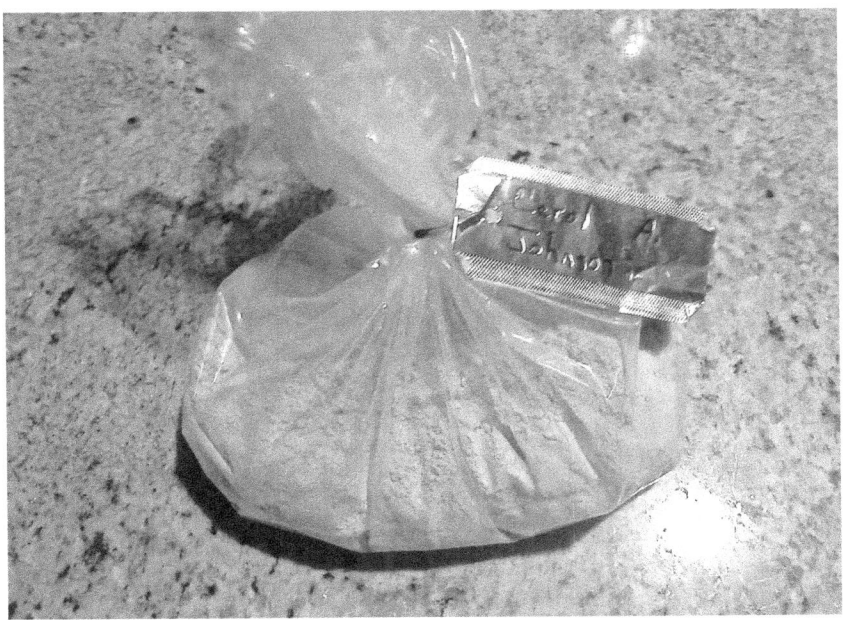

Time to open that box. Got me a little screwdriver, truth be told, took another Xanax, and I opened the box. I pulled out the plastic bag that contained the remains of my mother's physical self. I set it on the table and studied it for a moment. The first thing that popped into my head was a joke! I thought, she really looks pale! Then I had to look away for a moment because I knew the joke was a tactic to stop myself from crying in the moment. As I pulled away, the vision that came into my head was that last moment at Hospice Woodside that I looked at her physical body before I walked away, never to see her in that form again. I return my gaze onto the ashes left behind. As it sits, it begins to settle, which is actually quite 'unsettling' to me. As strange as it may sound, whenever at a funeral, I find myself staring at the chest of the deceased. Every time . . . I swear I see it moving. This person is not dead, is what I think to myself.

Janny and I decided that we are going to have our own personal memorial for her this Sunday, which will be her two week anniversary of her Re-Birth. We will spread some ashes on the beach. Then the following Sunday, we will have a larger memorial on the beach for others to attend. Al, her social worker from Hospice, will give her eulogy. Hope to see you there.

Love to all!!!

And life goes on . . . (2011-12-05 20:57) - Beth

It was my first day back to work today. I will admit, I was very apprehensive about returning. I've been gone for 4 months already, seems like just yesterday. I did take a Xanax when I got up in the morning because I was just so nervous that everyone would look at me with those sad, 'I'm so sorry' eyes and I just don't think I could have handled that. I just wanted to maintain and I did well. Although, those around me had much to do with that. My buddy, Dale, kinda made sure to spread the word . . . 'Don't be nice to me!'

I managed to get away with the day, basically, unscathed. It didn't really hit me until I got home. I felt so horrible for locking my little girl away when she has not really ever been alone for that amount of time. Through the fault of no one, she has been fortunate to have always had someone around to love her and for her to love. Let's face it, at this point, we pretty much know that she is as close to a little girl as I'm going to get. She's had a loss in her life also. She *loved* her Grammy back to health with the breast cancer!!! Anyway, she was still trembling after I had been home for a while. It just broke my heart.

Not to mention, the last time I came home from work, my mother was still here! This time . . . she wasn't. That was very sad to me! Other than my trembling dog, my house is empty . . .

Heeeeeeeere's Janny... (2011-12-15 08:55) - Janice

I have hesitated to blog, it just seemed like it was something special for Bethie and Louie (my nickname for Carol). Also, it's been so long since I've allowed myself to feel what I'm feeling. I've tried to stay strong, to go through the last three years clinically (you all know I think I'm a doctor). I have so many emotions running through my head at all times, I sometimes feel dizzy. But now I think I'm ready.

I feel sad that I don't have my Louie to talk to, to laugh with (and at), to cry with, to tell my secrets to, and to hear her secrets. She was my best friend and I miss her more than even I imagined I would.

I feel happy that she is at peace, with no pain or worries. She and I talked a lot about what we think Heaven is like and decided that each person's Heaven is different, that we will all spend eternity doing exactly what we want. She believed she would fly around all day eating strawberries. Louie couldn't wait to fly!!! Sometimes I think about her flying around and bouncing in the clouds, and I swear I hear that crazy laugh! I feel at peace knowing that she is up there on my side. We had a deal that when she got to Heaven, and she wants me to know she's with me, I would find a screw, as my nickname for her is Screwy Louie. So far, I've found three screws in very random places. Thanks for watching out for me, Louie!!!

I feel lost like I'm wandering around, not knowing what to do with myself. So much of the last three years were spent going to doctor's appointments, chemo (sometimes for eight hours or more), and, for the last five months, helping to care for her and just being there for her and Bethie. This was not a bad thing; I was also there for myself. I feel thankful that Louie, Bethie and I had that time. We've hit some rough spots in our relationships over the years and, at times, I think we all thought they would not be able to be repaired. That idea was put to rest on November 17, 2008. Since we found out about Louie's diagnosis of breast cancer, the three of us have been practically inseparable. Our relationships have not only been repaired, we came out of this period closer than we ever had been.

I feel blessed that I have found my Faith in God again. When I felt overwhelmed, I spoke to God and asked him to take my worries and problems from me, that I tried to carry them all and I am just not strong enough. Immediately, I felt physically lighter, as if a weight was lifted from my shoulders. I've never been much of a church person, and still am not, but I believe that anything is possible if you "give it to God" and really believe it.

I feel as if I'm rambling, and would like to finish up by saying something to my sister. Louie, I miss you, I miss your laugh, I miss your klutziness, I miss your silly sayings that we heard a mazillion times and that still cracked us up, I miss your hugs, and how you insisted that "we need I love you letters too" and how you could never remember what they were. When I think about you with my head, I am so relieved that you're in Heaven, hanging out with Mom, Daddy, Grandma Dixon, Ed, and Justin, eating Gram's peanut butter fudge. When I think about you with my heart, I feel an emptiness inside that I don't believe will ever be able to be filled again. And I want to thank you and Bethie for allowing me into your home, your lives and your hearts. The time I spent with you is one of the most precious memories I have and I will carry that with me until we meet again in Heaven. Fly free and rest well, my sister, my friend, my hero. I love you!!!

Happy Birthday, My Angel! (2011-12-19 20:27) - Beth

Yes, today would have been my mother's 64th birthday. She told me once that she thought everyone in heaven was in their 30's. So perhaps, she turned 34 today in her heaven. Today was pretty difficult for me, for instance, I just typed three lines and had to stop to cry for my mother. I miss her SO much! It's so different coming home to an empty house . . . just my little Roxy who is trembling and dehydrated from her separation anxiety. For a long time, I would come home from work and kiss my mother and play with my overly joyous puppy cause she hung out with Grammy all day. Ma would be up preparing dinner. We would make jokes that I was the man and she was the woman. I would be the one out working, putting air in the tires and fixing the roof and she would be the one who stayed home, cared for the puppy and prepared dinner. Those were the good old days. I really miss those days! Today kind of crept up on me too. I wasn't thinking yesterday, 'Boy tomorrow is going to be hard for me because it's her birthday.' I had to leave the office several times today because my emotions were getting to me and I hate to cry in front of people. Plus, I'm still fearful I'm going to just lose it one of these days either by having a nervous breakdown or end up killing someone. You know, when good daughters go bad, kind of thing.

Now, I'm worried about tomorrow because that is her one month anniversary of her 'Re-Birth'. How will I handle that? I never realized until today that she was born on the 19th and passed on the 20th. Does that mean I'm going to mourn both of those days all the time? Is it weird that I carry my mom's ashes around with me if I feel the need to be physically close to her? I know she's here spiritually, but sometimes I need that physical closeness. That's another weird thing . . . sometimes I'll stare at her ashes and then I pull up the last image ever taken of her after she had passed and it just amazes me and terrifies me all at the same time. You can actually feel fragments of bone matter. Sometimes when I place my hand on the bag, it feels as if she is holding my hand. It's kind of soothing. But is that weird? I don't know. I've never been through anything like this in my life.

Last night I decided to put the Christmas tree up. 'Our' tradition was to put it up on her birthday. I, however, need to create new traditions. Plus, I thought it would be too difficult to do the same tradition without her. It was still very hard on my heart. My mother wasn't much for Christmas for many years. Then something changed . . . I think I persuaded her to appreciate it. From then on, every year she bought me something relating to Christmas. She bought 24 karat gold ornaments for years . . . enough to cover my entire tree. Then, of course, the gold star for the top. It's beautiful, but not the same without her!

We held her memorial at the beach in Treasure Island on December 11th. It was very intimate with around 20 people or so. Janny brought 3 dozen balloons in pink and purple in color. Al (Ma's social worker, and NO he can't be 'friends' with us for 18 months or something ridiculous, just sayin') was prepared to give her eulogy. He was wonderful! We laughed, we cried . . . so cliché, but true. I felt like I literally had a nervous breakdown that day, all day! I could not stop trembling. It scared me. I was very glad that I had Janny at my side holding my hand. I think I may have paid her back from when she was having labor pains with my little Twinkie-Head. I believe I was squeezing her hand pretty hard! Sorry, Janny.

Wow, this has been a very long blog so I think I will create a new blog entitled 'The Eulogy' because it's pretty long too.

Thanks for following along and love to all!

The Eulogy (2011-12-19 20:48) - Beth

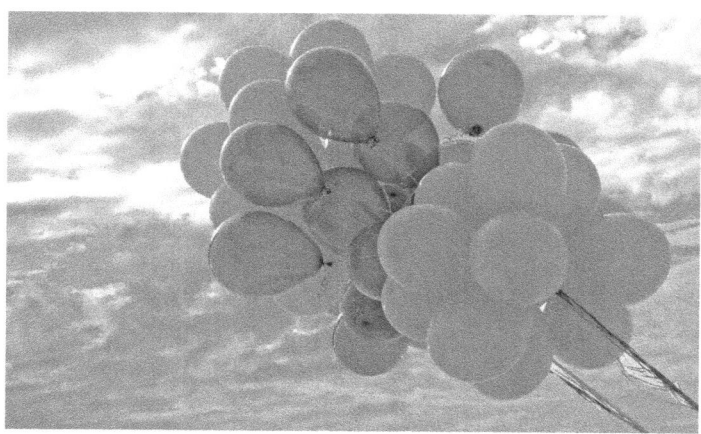

My name is Al Perrone, and I had the privilege of being Carol's counselor in the last year of her life. At Suncoast Hospice, we are told that every person we assist is equal, and we should treat each person with the same level of attention and respect. That being said, we're not supposed to have "favorites". I can say to all of you now, that I broke that rule when I met Carol Johnson. I met Carol a year ago yesterday, on December 10, 2010, at her home following admission to our team.

The first thing I remember about walking up to her house was the patio. The house, with its Sienna and terra cotta finish, was complemented by a deep blue ornate column holding up the patio awning. I remember thinking how this was something that stands out in a crowd and isn't expected. How ironic that a few moments later, I would be meeting a lady I could describe with similar words. The next thing I remember was barking. As I knocked on the door, I instantly heard Roxy letting me know that she was here and was going to protect her granny. Carol answered the door. She was small in stature, with a smile bigger than life. I began talking with Carol and Beth about what my role would be in her care, and I started to get to know these ladies. Over that first hour, I learned about Carol's life. I picked up on her Pennsylvanian accent almost immediately and we talked about her life prior to her illness, her hobbies, including puzzles, and her love for her family, in particular, Beth and Janice.

She and Beth asked me many questions that day, and there was a sense of intense listening I distinctly remember feeling. With each question the family asked, there seemed to be a sense of relief, a sense that some of the fears they had with Hospice coming into their home had washed away a little. I remember joking with Carol and Beth and feeling my sense of humor and personality meshed so well with theirs. Then, in explaining the hospice philosophy, I said three words that would come back to haunt Beth and Janice for the next year. I told Carol, "You're the boss." Over the next 11 months, anytime Carol did not want to do something, she need only look at her sister and daughter and say, "Al said I'm the boss, so no." The visit took longer than I had expected it to (gladly), and I went on my way, thinking that I had made a real connection with a family and looked forward to working for them.

This would be the part in the relationship where Carol started playing "Hard to get." Carol would cancel appointments early on, or reschedule them, or leave me to drive Roxy crazy by knocking on the door repeatedly. I would occasionally make it into the house, eventually meeting Janice, but the visits would often be met with answering questions, getting to know each other a little more, laughing and then weeks of no contact. Any other family, this would have been a bigger deal, but there was something about Carol that allowed me to be ok with it. With Carol, I knew that patience was key. When she was ready, she would let me know. Pushing her to talk would do no good. And eventually, she was ready.

Beth asked me to come to the house. Her mother was ready to make some decisions. Carol, Beth, and Janice were all present, and I feel THAT was truly when this wonderful relationship, I will always treasure, began to flourish. These three wonderful people welcomed me into their homes, into their lives and allowed me to see who they all truly are. Carol, vulnerable, funny and kind. Beth, determined, funny and creative. Janice, clever, funny and tenacious. Can you tell there was a lot of funny in that house?

I distinctly remember watching a "back and forth" between Carol and Beth about Carol's "stupid looking hats" she would wear when she was growing her hair back. I think all three of them must have said "stupid looking hats" about 20 times that day. The family also got a lot of mileage out of my inability to open their front door correctly. I think I FINALLY got the hang of that deadbolt one of the last times I was in their home.

Over the next few months, Carol decided, with some soul searching, that she was done with treatment to extend her life. She felt it more important that her life have quality in its last few months, because, after all, she was the boss.

As she began to decline, Janice moved in, and the relationship between these three women changed and grew even stronger. I think part of the reason I liked going to their home as much as I did was that in many ways it felt like a television sitcom in some ways. You had very three distinct, complementary personalities living together (four if you count Roxy) in a house and above everything else, from tensions to laughter, from frustration to snarky humor, there was love apparent. Janice and Beth, you created a wonderful, beautiful environment for Carol to spend her final months in. The two of you worked so beautifully together. Know that you did Carol proud in your care of her. She told me on multiple occasions how lucky she was to have you as her annoying cheerleaders, always willing to take care of whatever she needed, if that need was a kick in the pants every once in a while.

Over the summer, we saw a decline in Carol. She was becoming weaker and more confused. We thought that it was getting close to the end and our continuous care staff was called in to assist Carol to make the transition to the next plane. Our CC staff will usually be in a home for a day or two, maybe three. **THREE WEEKS** later, Carol rebounded. Carol's team - Lori, Terri and I - would have conversations where we could not figure out what was keeping Carol going. We all forgot a very important piece of the puzzle. Carol was the boss. She wasn't ready yet.

It was during those weeks that I had one of the most profound moments of my professional career, and I have Carol to thank for that. I was sitting on a chair by Carol's bedside, holding her hand, and she asked me about the dying process, what it was like. I told her that everyone dies differently. She asked me what I thought it was going to be like when she died. Talk about putting me on the spot.

I told her that I felt that people died the way they lived and that she struck me as a person who always tried to live with class, beauty and dignity, and when it was her time, she would pass with class, beauty and dignity. She cried a little, said she hoped so, and sent me out of the room, but not before telling me she loved me. And I loved her, too. I still do.

There are some memories in the last few months of Carol's life that many of us here would choose to gladly forget. There are, however, some memories in that time I will cherish. The stories that Beth and Janice shared with me while Carol rested in her room. Helping Carol to see the love and affection she was experiencing around her. Throwing the chew toy for Roxy while talking with the family. But if there is one memory I will always hold dear, it would be during one of my last visits where, in helping Carol to move from her bedroom to the living room, she started to dance with me. She was so fragile I was scared that she would fall, but she seemed, in that brief moment, happy. She was smiling and laughing. She is the only patient I have ever danced with. She's also the only patient I have ever had grab my butt immediately following the dance. But that's just the kinda girl Carol was. And that's why we love her.

The last time I saw Carol she was moving to our Woodside facility. I would look at our morning report every morning hoping that Carol had transcended, knowing that this is what she wanted, that she was ready. She had to only wait for God to finish her apartment in Heaven. And on a Sunday afternoon, God brought Carol home. As to what Carol's Heaven might be like, I think she summed it up best on October 22, 2010, when she wrote: "As I stepped outside this morning I was magically transported back to a day...many days...in my childhood. It was a beautiful day, the sky a gorgeous blue with soft, billowy clouds, birds chirping. It reminded me of a summer day in the little town of New Brighton many years ago and I pictured myself hopping out of bed, hands and face washed, teeth brushed, hair combed, dressed, bed made and ready to run out the door with a piece of toast in hand to meet my friends. We would play hopscotch, ride bikes, play hide & seek till lunchtime. Our moms never minded packing us a picnic lunch to have under the neighbor's 'snowball bush', which also served as a cottage or a cave or a hiding place from the 'stupid' boys, depending on our whim. In the afternoons we might play paper dolls on someone's porch or look for pictures in the clouds or roll down the hill over and over again, just because it was fun. When our dads came home from work, it was supper time, then baths, put on your pj's and catch lightning bugs."

I miss Carol a lot, as all of us do. She was, in many ways, a force to be reckoned with, and in others, a fragile soul that needed to be sheltered. I will never forget her smile, her voice, and her tears.

Carol enjoyed working on puzzles in the year that I knew her. In many ways, Carol was looking for the final piece to the puzzle in her life, but it was God who found it and made her complete.

Christmas without her . . . (2011-12-26 20:13) - Beth

Tuesday, December 20th

I went shopping for those pesky things that I couldn't order online. I am trying to think on a really personal level, what the people on my Christmas list would want. I am excited about the things that I am giving this year! However, it is very sad that my mom had always been my goal for Christmas to create the best Christmas for her, ever. If she cried (in a good way), I did my job! She has been through so much bullshit in her life that I just wanted to do everything I could to make her happy that one time a year. She deserved that . . .

Janny & I decided to go through some of her stained glass and gift it to those deserving . . . you will soon know who you are. My mother loved each of you dearly. And I thank you for giving her that gift of love. She loved Lori; she always perked up when Lori entered the room! Thank you, Lori!!!

She loved Al; she canceled a lot of appointments with him, but ultimately . . . she loved him! She thought of him as 'Schmit, II'. Just as he mentioned in the eulogy and she did the same with 'JoeCastro' (one word), she had more disco in her that she HAD to get out of her system. She even grabbed Al's ass when the dance was over.

It is very sad to me that I am not gifting anything to my mother this year. She's not here. I have a sneaking suspicion that I may sit in front of the Christmas tree on Christmas morning . . . mourning! I think I will cry for a long time and then; hopefully, I will feel better. There are new things I will experience in my 'new' lifetime that will continue to grow me as a person.

I wonder if you are feeling particularly lonely and missing your best friend if you can actually 'feel' that in your heart. Cause I gotta tell ya, my heart hurts so bad!!

Friday, December 23rd

It was time to make the homemade chicken noodle soup that I hold so fondly in my heart as it was one of our many traditions. This was one of the hardest traditions to 'get over' actually! She missed it last year as well because she slept through the entire process. Thank God I had a friend over, Dale, to exchange gifts and he ended up helping me last year. This year, knowing that my mother wouldn't be here to help, Dale offered his assistance again. And thankfully, I accepted. What a process that turned out to be!

Before we even began, I pondered the fact that my Grandpap would always be responsible for my dough shrinking back after I roll it out and I wondered if he and my mother would get their silly heads together and play jokes on me. Turns out . . . they did! And my Grandpap was up there laughing with his belly shaking like a bowl full of jelly - yet not making a sound . . . then my mother's uproarious laughter that magically makes the whole room laugh.

Anyway, here's the joke . . . they apparently thought it would be funny to make me mix cement with my bare hands! That is what it felt like. I have been making these noodles probably around 25 years and it has been impossible to add too much flour. Impossible! This year . . . added too much flour. Had already started with 18 eggs; ended up adding 3 more for a grand total of 21 eggs. I literally, pulled a muscle in my boob by mixing this concrete. I almost threw it out thinking, this is not going to be good. Ended up rolling up a batch to boil and try out. Turns out they are as yummy as ever and I wish Ma had a chance to try them, even though she was up there cackling at me!

Thank you again for your help, Dale!

Saturday, December 24th

Had to make the meatballs today. My hands and upper body were so sore from mixing those noodles last night. Damn concrete! Anyway, had to suffer through it . . . it's for Janny. So,

I did. As I'm mixing, I notice that the consistency isn't what it normally is and these aren't going to turn out. Almost threw it out, but I didn't.

Going to Janny's for Christmas Eve. Can't decide whether or not to take Roxy with me. I really want to get her more socialized, but I am also still trying to get me more socialized. I cannot deal with her inhibitions about meeting others and going different places if I am still working on that myself. I'm trying to do this 'WITH' her. When I think about how social I used to be, it really shocks me to find myself in this mindset. I really just want to be alone for the most part even though I know that is not healthy for me. I'm working on that. So, I took her!

I got choked up on the way over because last year my mother was in the passenger seat with Roxy on her lap. My big alligator tears were blurring my vision and I was trying to drive. Note to self: Don't let friends drive crying! Anyway, I got through the evening and it was very nice. Roxy was a pretty good girl too. She is getting more social.

I arrived home and lit my ceramic bags that my mom bought me that lights a trail to your house for Santa to follow. Another one of our traditions. They blew out quickly. For some reason, they usually do.

Sunday, December 25th

I wanted to sleep until I woke up on my own. Since I have a dog and not a kid, that wasn't really much of a problem. We got up at 11 am. I put the soup on, the meatballs, turned on the tree lights and had a mimosa. That's what my mother and I always did. We would always put Elvis' Christmas album on for decorating and opening gifts. I haven't been able to listen to that CD this year at all.

Had to finish wrapping Roxy's gifts in the morning. She is jumping up to the studio table wanting to retrieve them; however, she's only knee-high to a grasshopper. I am such a bad momma. Maybe this is why God won't let me have kids of my own. I should have had those wrapped before now.

Janny and Joe came over and brought the family. It was a nice visit and I received very thoughtful gifts. LC got me one of those 'clean smelling' candles. I love those. And Joe got me men's cleaning supplies as I can even 'fix you woof up there'. Janny got me a necklace that will hold some of my mother's ashes. She didn't even prepare me for that. At least I took her aside for the gift that I knew would make her cry. That's just the kinda girl she is. Eventually, I gave them the 'sign' that we gave to my mom when she wanted us to leave and it worked . . . they left. I cleaned up the kitchen and took a nap . . . until 11 pm. Haaaa. I got up to give Roxy her snack and realized, I never ate any soup or meatballs. Decided I would have a nice bowl of soup and that's what I did. And then I went to bed, again.

I was just glad I got through it without a breakdown. Perhaps that is what I need ultimately, but I want to be the one to predict when that is going to be. Trying to show some self-control.

Anyway . . . that was my Christmas without her!

I miss you SO much and I love you with ALL my heart!!!

From Bad Day to Sad Day (2011-12-29 20:49) - Beth

Started by having a bad day at work. I have got to get out of there! I have never seen so many disrespectful people in my life, and **this** is management. Everything is a secret, including what our hours are and weekends that we are *required* to work being notified about 12 hours in advance. They actually made employees decide between their Christmas bonuses or their (already approved) personal time off during the holidays and just give up that time that they earned! Who does that? They want to know that they are the 'Puppet Masters'. They dangle the carrot and then just rip it away again. That is intolerable to me. Being in a position of 'power' does not give you the right to be disrespectful. I've been a business owner and I know, **having** been in the position of power, you lead by example!

I have a small amount of insurance money coming and I am seriously thinking about quitting and doing my own thing again. I have several wonderful ideas that I've been kicking around way too long and I really need to make them my reality. And all of them will benefit many wonderful people that just need a little help. My mom always worried that I had too much ambition for 'saving the world' being afraid that I would be disappointed if I didn't, but I always told her, 'I can save the world by saving one person at a time. That person will help someone else. And that person will help someone.' I believe I have **that** power. I believe we ALL have that power!

So upon arriving home, I just really missed my mom. It was so nice that when I used to have a bad day, I could come home and know that I had someone to listen to me vent. Or a shoulder to cry on. She was always in my corner and that always made me feel better! I really miss her.

I had to get into my shed to grab my cooler for a stupid potluck that we're having at the stupid office that I didn't want to partake in to begin with until someone came over and suggested I bring a cooler. Fine, whatever. So, I decided to rinse it out with the hose and when I opened the hose reel I looked down and found a perfectly shaped heart leaf. That is one of the signs that my mother was going to give me when she was there with me because ever since I was a little girl, I used to find random heart shaped rocks and I would always bring them home to my mom because she was *always* my heart! That made me feel a little better. I've inherited that heart collection now and am adding to it with the many hearts that I'm finding around me. I haven't completed cleaning out her room. I seem to go in for a while and then run across something that makes it too hard to keep going. Tonight I walked in and the first thing I saw was her birth certificate and then I saw the wig that she just looked so damn cute in, and I was out. I would really just like to get that done before the 1st of 2012!

I am so ready to say goodbye to 2011. This was without a doubt **the** most painful year of my life! I am ready to move forward. I am prepared to show my Ma, as she flies around up there, that I CAN change the world and I'm ready to go . . . balls to the wall!!! And I'm also ready to show the world that **they** can make a difference too with very little effort on their part. It's amazing all the good we could do in this world if we all worked together. I'm ready to change that.

Bring it . . . 2012. I'm ready for ya!!!

Dear 2011, (2011-12-30 19:10) - Beth

First and foremost, I would like to thank you for the tender, precious moments that you allowed me to have with my mother during your year. I will hold onto those memories forever!

However, I have chosen to say 'Goodbye' to other moments that I don't care to hold onto any longer during your year. I would like to start with GUILT.

~ the guilt I had for not being there for my mother every time she fell so I could prevent it. Goodbye.

~ the guilt I had when I felt the need to get away from it all for a bit or I was going to lose my mind. Goodbye.

~ the guilt I had when she was so sick and there was nothing I could do to help her. Goodbye.

~ the guilt I had for being forced to go back to work for financial purposes and couldn't attend every appointment with her any longer. Goodbye.

~ the guilt I had every morning when I would tell her goodbye and then to walk out that door and leave her to go to work. Goodbye.

~ the guilt I had that I hadn't spent the night with her on November 19th. Goodbye.

~ the guilt I had when I found myself frustrated that when I was running an errand for my mom and she would describe step by step exactly how she wanted it done and where I was to do it. Goodbye.

~ the guilt for not, in general, being MORE present in the here and now. Goodbye.

I would also like to say Goodbye to those 'not so precious' flashback moments that have been replaying in my mind over and over again.

~ that very last breath that she took, that took my breath away! As precious as it was, it was also most heart-wrenching! It was such a bittersweet moment for me. I knew she wanted to go and she wanted her family around her. She had both; however, at the same time, I was losing my mother and best friend!!! Goodbye.

(Oddly enough, I reach into the pocket of my mother's robe that I am wearing. It's the only thing left that I haven't washed yet. I find a paper towel. I use it to wipe away the tears that are blurring my vision when it dawns on me that she probably used that very paper towel to wipe away tears of her own. Wow, profound.)

~ when she fell and I was the one that was helping her to the bathroom. Goodbye.

~ when I walk out the French doors and remember that Ma grabbed the mask to break out. Goodbye.

~ when my own Mother called me a 'lying bitch' when I told her, 'I am your daughter!' I know it wasn't her, but somehow . . . that doesn't make it feel any better. Goodbye.

~ when my Ma yelled out the window, 'Help'. It was so pathetic and sad. She could barely even yell, but she wanted to throw that vase out the window to escape. Goodbye.

~ and to all the other bad moments that continue to fill my mind. Goodbye.

I choose to let those memories go at the end of your year and only focus on the pleasant memories and place the rest of my mind on my goals to make things happen for myself in the coming year!

Helpless No More, Beth

Dear 2012,

Welcome to my life. I have a lot of wonderful things planned during your term. Would greatly appreciate any & all guidance you are able to offer. I fully embrace you!

Enthusiastically yours, Beth

2012 January

I especially miss her today . . .
(2012-01-05 19:43) - Beth

I miss my mother every day; however, I especially miss her today . . . I've been trying really hard to hold to my 'Goodbye 2011' promise to myself. I've been doing very well, in my opinion. I placed my mom in her 'temporary' hangout (undisturbed) on the 2nd of January until I can figure some things out for permanent placement and I have left her there to rest rather than continue to carry her around because I need that physical closeness. Today I felt the need for that. I miss coming home and embracing her! I know that I can speak to her and she will hear me, but sometimes . . . I just miss the physical aspects of having her here with me. I haven't gotten her out and I hope to fight the urge.

I especially miss her today; at work, I became overwhelmed with the saddest memories of the past year. As much as I tried to force them away . . . they weren't going anywhere. I had to fight past the tears; staring at the computer screen. I took several deep breaths and I am pleased to announce that I fought my way through it without any Xanax even. I love that!

Once I arrived home, I thought about the funny, happy memories of that silly lady and it made me laugh and cry at the same time. How does that happen? I don't expect to not have any bad moments in the next few years of missing my mother, but I also don't want to just become a hermit or some weird artist that just produces this really freaky artwork that nobody even understands. Including the artist him/herself!

Therefore, my goal is to focus ALL my energy on my projects that I've come up with during this entire process from fighting breast cancer to battling pancreatic cancer. She is a warrior! She is my HERO!!!

<u>*I PROMISE TO MAKE HER PROUD!*</u>

'Today I am grateful . . . ' (2012-01-08 19:26) - Beth

In the continuing effort in cleaning out Ma's room (it's a process, sometimes you just have to walk away), I found several pages of dated 'Today I am grateful . . .' I believe this is a project that Dr. Shrink gave to her. I thought it was pretty cute and enjoyed reading it. I chose to share it with you all.

4/28/09 - Today I am grateful . . .
for my precious daughter, Beth, who takes such good care of me
for our little dog, Roxy, who makes me laugh
for my sister, Janice, & the relationship we have
4/29 - Today I am grateful . . .
for the smell of orange blossoms
for the sunshine on my face
for a phone call from one of my dearest friends, Rick
4/30 - Today I am grateful . . .
for the smell of orange blossoms

for the sunshine on my face
for a phone call from one of my dearest friends, Rick
5/1 - Today I am grateful . . .
that we sold the plotter & can pay another month's mortgage
that Ken's foundation may want to do a benefit golf outing for project, 'I am Beautiful'
for my precious daughter, Beth
5/2 - Today I am grateful . . .
that I got all green lights from 13th Ave to 46th Ave
that we got a gas card from the American Cancer Society
that Beth's friend took her out & got her mind off things for a while
5/3 - Today I am grateful . . .
for cuddling on the couch with little Roxy
5/4 - Today I am grateful . . .
that Cindy's surgery went well
for 'The Memory Vase'
5/5 - Today I am grateful . . .
for the smell of roses when Gramma is here
5/6 - Today I am grateful . . .
for 'girls' night in'.
5/7 - Today I am grateful . . .
that the tumor is shrinking significantly
for a Mother's Day card from Marie
for a nice dinner with Beth
5/8 - Today I am grateful . . .
for no Neulasta
for a Mother's Day card from Lisa, James & kids
that Beth makes every day Mother's Day

5/9 - Today I am grateful...
for a Mother's Day card from Mom
that John & Cindy made it back to Oklahoma okay
for meds that help me sleep through the pain
5/10 - Today I am grateful...
for Beth, the reason Mother's Day has meaning
for a phone call from Rick
for a phone call from John
5/11 - Today I am grateful...
that I didn't cry at my appointment with Dr. Shrink
for a check from Beth's dad
5/12 - Today I am grateful...
for a call from Mom
5/15 - Today I am grateful...
for hugs from Dr. S
5/17 - Today I am grateful...
for a great night's sleep
for a beautiful day
for making brunch for Beth & Jan
5/18 - Today I am grateful...
for a $125 grant from CancerCare
5/19 - Today I am grateful...
for sleeping pills
5/20 - Today I am grateful...
that Beth made meatballs for girls' night in
for laughs with Beth & Janice
5/21 - Today I am grateful...
that John's surgery went well
for 1/2 dose of Taxol
that my hemoglobin count is getting back to normal

5/22 - Today I am grateful . . .
that I'm able to return my shopping cart to the store
for a rainy day
for a long nap
5/23 - Today I am grateful . . .
that Beth went out & had fun
for Auntie Ann's sesame pretzels
for a letter from the IRS
5/24 - Today I am grateful . . .
for less bone & joint pain
5/25 - Today I am grateful . . .
that John continues to improve
5/26 - Today I am grateful . . .
for a nice conversation with a woman in line at the bank
for help from a nice woman at Health & Human Services
5/27 - Today I am grateful . . .
for a very nice voicemail from my dear friend/mentor, Bob
for a (scary) conversation & hug from a cancer patient
for an impromptu girls' night in
(pretty much the only laughs today)
5/28 - Today I am grateful . . .
for a conversation with a cancer (colon, liver, lungs)
patient at chemo
for a nice lunch with Beth & Janice (Jan's treat)
for unexpectedly seeing & getting a big hug from
brother-in-law, Joe G
hemoglobin continues to rise to normal
for Mom having a birthday cake for breakfast
with Dad, Gram & Ed

5/29 - Today I am grateful...
for $300 from Human Services
for a check from Beth's dad
5/30 - Today I am grateful...
that I decided to have the surgery
that Beth & Janice got pink ribbon tattoos in my honor
that I have such a large support group of family & friends
5/31 - Today I am grateful...
for a really long nap
6/1 - Today I am grateful...
that I felt well enough to get some work done
that I was tired for a reason!
6/2 - Today I am grateful...
for feeling good
for a delicious girls' night in dinner
for laughs with Beth, Jan & Roxy
6/3 - Today I am grateful...
that I felt well enough to bake goodies for the chemo nurses
6/4 - Today I am grateful...
that Lauren went to chemo with us
that my liver enzymes & blood work are good
that Jan took us for a nice lunch
6/5 - Today I am grateful...
for very little pain
6/6 - Today I am grateful...
for a care package from Janice
for no need to take pain pills
6/7 - Today I am grateful...
for a long overdue call from brother Joe
that Heidi is doing better

6/8 - Today I am grateful . . .
for a card & check from Dennis & Michelle
John continues to make progress
Cindy is well enough to return to work
6/9 - Today I am grateful . . .
for a nice phone conversation with my friend/mentor, Bob
for another fun girls' night in
that I am feeling pretty good

That's where it ended. I chose to believe that's when she ended the project, not because she didn't have anything to be grateful for after June 9th, 2009! I love and miss her every day!!!

Bursting with Excitement . . .
(2012-01-10 19:38) - Beth

Oh my goodness, I just took a huge leap today. I turned in my resignation. My last day will be January 20th. My birthday is January 21st, Happy Birthday to me!

Don't get me wrong, I didn't just quit my job all willy-nilly without thoroughly thinking through this entire plan. I made the commitment to work on all of the projects that were inspired by my mother that will help countless people during difficult times. I am so passionate about each and every one of them. Failure is not an option!

Now, as I sit here all giddy like a little girl in a candy store, my mind is flooding with 'Holy crap, you have a million things to do!' What will I work on first? I have to come up with a solid plan for each of my ideas. This will be my full-time job.

I just told Janny last night that I hadn't heard the song 'Satisfied' that I posted on a previous blog since my mother passed. I heard that song multiple times a day when Ma was still here. Today, shortly after I turned in my resignation, that song played on Pandora. Made me believe I made the right decision!

So, I'm wondering if I should start a new blog, beings this is the start of a whole new journey . . . a new lifestyle. I could call it 'One Woman 1 Mission . . . to save the world'. I like that. Or should I just start a new chapter on the same blog? Taking votes on this one.

The two projects that I want to begin with because I believe I can do this very low budget but with huge success! That is the 'Drain Necklace' and 'Second Chance'

The 'Drain Necklace' is a medical accessory, if you will. It aids women in dealing with the drains that are inserted into their sides to drain the lymphatic fluids after a mastectomy. Long story, but I will keep you posted on all happenings on this project. I am hoping to obtain a licensing deal with Jackson Pratt on this product since they already have the clientele.

'Second Chance' is the pilot reality show that I want to shoot where in each episode, one displaced family will be taken off the streets and given all that is needed to get their lives back in order for 6 to 12 months before they are completely back on their own.

I am so excited to begin now that I've made the commitment. Oh, I've also made the commitment to myself and Roxy that we are going to start getting way more exercise. Yes, I'm thin and always have been, but not really that healthy. Also, I'm going to be forced to become more social again. I have to mingle with people to complete my projects. I am confident you will be seeing me on the news and in the papers. Might be nice if I met my dream man somewhere along the way! Funny story, I had a dream the other night and met a guy. I was pretty attracted to him and thought, yeah, maybe. Turns out, he was a loser. I can't even dream of my own dream man. What the hell . . .

That's all for now folks. Thanks for following along. Love you all, mean it!

Her Car's gone now . . . (2012-01-16 19:11) - Beth

I sold her car to an acquaintance of mine. He owns a used car lot. It was bittersweet. I was glad that it was sold and the last of her physical being in a large format has been eliminated, but it's lived here for the last eleven years. It's really weird to look out the kitchen window and not see her car there.

She had a really difficult time giving up her car when I mentioned selling it previously but she was heavily narcotized. Turns out, I didn't sell it until almost two months after she passed. I'm very sorry that I put her through that worry early on.

I miss her very much every day! I am ready to dive into the projects that she was the inspiration behind, which is all of them. I am a little overwhelmed, but I will figure it out. I don't want to just work on one project at a time. I have too much going on for that. Plus, I plan to sell some of my ideas out-right so I can begin on the next projects!!!

C'mon, I'm looking for opinions on whether or not to start a new blog or continue with a new chapter.

Only two more days . . . (2012-01-18 18:24) - Beth

Only two more days before my life is turned back over to **me**. No longer predicted by anyone else. No one to blame . . . but me. No one to credit . . . but me. I am so ready for this challenge! I actually, look quite forward to it. I'm anxious to introduce my projects to open arms and I think this is the perfect time for all of them. I created 'Second Chance' in 2007 and took it nowhere. I guess it just wasn't the right time then. NOW is the time!

The awesome news **is** that I already have my first sponsor for 'Second Chance'. My dentist was one that I wanted to discuss sponsorship with. I decided that since I am losing my benefits (the only **con** I came up with while determining whether or not to go out on my own), I better at least get my teeth cleaned! I simply told him what I was getting into and asked if he would consider being the dental sponsor for my displaced family. He committed, **just like that**. Some think that this is going to be a very costly project, but apparently, they don't get the idea. I am looking for everything to be **donated** to this family. I think it is going to be very challenging for me to put this all together, but I believe it is going to be a huge success and worth every effort!

I am about to place ALL my fears to the side and show people exactly what I am capable of. I NEED to make a difference in peoples' lives or life just isn't worth living. I was put here for a purpose and I need to explore all my ideas to find out which one it is.

When my mother was diagnosed with breast cancer, she and I seriously discussed suicide. I knew she was ready as she was so against any type of treatment and I really believed I could **NOT** live without her. Something continued to hold me back. I felt that I had been placed here for a reason. I have something left to do. Something left to give. I couldn't do it.

All of this is in honor of my mother! If I'm not doing something meaningful, I would rather not be here. That is why I chose to quit my hum-drum boring job that a monkey could do . . . to make a difference or die trying!

That's all I have.

End of This Chapter . . . (2012-01-22 21:41) - Beth

This is the end of this chapter. My mother was reborn on the 20th of November. I was reborn on the 21st of January. I am ready for this new chapter of my life. The chapter that I either go hard or go home! I really feel that if I'm not doing what I was placed here to do, then I am not doing my life justice and I might as well pack it up.

I decided that tonight was the night to burn the 'Comfort Candle'. It looked so beautiful burning there with her remains beneath it. I did have to reach into the box with which I placed her just to be closer to her for a minute. But then I moved on!

I am going to end this story and begin another. I am going to take the inspiration from my mother and take it to the next level. She was my biggest fan and I know that she still is. Please continue to follow along. I will not let you all down! The time starts now . . .

> Anonymous (2012-01-24 22:41:09)
> Look out world, the Beth Pauvlinch that I saw develop from a scrawny, carefree teenager into a CEO, an Artist, an ever-loving person (that now writes better than me - - I know, not saying much) is back in life's saddle and wanting to take us all for a ride. Hold on tight, it is going to be a helluva ride.
> I love you and cannot wait to see where you take us this time.

Be careful but never stop being Beth.
Mike

2012 August

One final sentiment . . . (2012-08-25 18:34) - Beth

I believe I mentioned several times in this blog about the rose that my cousin's boyfriend brought to my mother one day months before she passed. It was the most aromatic rose I had ever smelled. I actually accused him of dousing it with some type of perfume.

That rose grew weary, turned brown and passed well before my mother; however, that rose continued to smell beautiful with not a drop of water in all these months.

I just smelled that rose and it no longer has the fragrance that continued to drag me into my mother's room (I left it for her) even after her passing. I wondered for a moment what that possibly could mean. It made me sad for a moment and then I determined why I would choose to believe it no longer carried that fabulous aroma. I believe it means . . . my mother's rose garden in heaven has now blossomed!

I love you and miss you more than you will ever know! Enjoy your rose garden!

MEET THE AUTHORS

Carol 'CJ' Johnson

Carol lived a rather rough life. She had Beth pretty young and was single. Some family members encouraged her to adopt Beth out; she refused. She struggled financially while raising her but she NEVER gave up. They became very close when Beth was young.

Beth was terribly saddened when she learned that Carol had cancer and would have the biggest battle of her life. But Carol just put her big girl panties on, and gave one hell of a fight! She is truly Beth's hero!

Beth Pauvlinch

I began my creative journey dating back to the age of eight by creating a crayon drawn book for my mother. I cut up an old pair of my favorite boots to use as the cover. As she looked through it, she cried tears of joy. From that point forward, I vowed to challenge myself with every gift I gave her. I wanted to see those tears of joy every time I gifted her. My mother has been my biggest inspiration in following my dreams and my heart.

www.ingramcontent.com/pod-product-compliance
Lightning Source LLC
Chambersburg PA
CBHW052133010526
44113CB00035B/2023